Reality and/or Realities

Reality and/or Realities

MAURICIO ABADI
AND
SUSAN HALE ROGERS

WITH A CONTRIBUTION BY NOÉ JITRIK

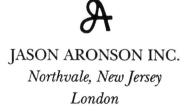

JASON ARONSON INC.
Northvale, New Jersey
London

This book was set in 12 pt. Baskerville by Alpha Graphics of Pittsfield, N.H. and printed and bound by Haddon Craftsmen of Scranton, Pennsylvania.

Library of Congress Cataloging-in-Publication Data

Abadi, Mauricio.
    Reality and/or realities / by Mauricio Abadi and Susan Rogers.
      p. cm.
    Includes bibliographical references and index.
    ISBN 1-56821-536-3 (hardcover : alk. paper)
    1. Reconstruction (Psychoanalysis) 2. Psychoanalytic
interpretation. 3. Representation (Psychoanalysis) 4. Reality.
    I. Rogers, Susan (Susan Hale) II. Title.
    RC489.R39A23   1995
    150.19'5—dc20   95-5895

Manufactured in the United States of America. Jason Aronson Inc. offers books and cassettes. For information and catalog write to Jason Aronson Inc., 230 Livingston Street, Northvale, New Jersey 07647.

"Reality is a failed imitation of myth"
Mauricio Abadi

Contents

1

Construction:
Between History and Myth

Mauricio Abadi

"A memory is a bit of eternity."
      —Antonio Porchia

"A bit of eternity is already all eternity."
      —Macedonio Fernandez

To Evemere, perseverant in his error. He believed that the myth was born of a succession of distortions of history, and so he ignored that history is an obstinate attempt (recurrently failed) to realize and to materialize the myth. My long dialogue with him did allow me, however, to salvage the implicit value of his manifest mistake: without the historical (the preconscious material), the myth (the ineffable unconscious) could never reach the epiphany of the verb: "Tell me your history and I'll tell you your myth."

The Mirage of History

Bi-frontal Janus. His two faces. Retrospection and prospection. Looking back in order to look ahead. Discovering, through a looking-glass, that the mirror is reflecting what happens later. Constructing a model of a supposed past in order to account for a rite that makes it eternal: the symptom. Construction (as a detective constructs) of a myth, the foundation of the commemorative liturgy of the symptom. The structure of the symptom endlessly repeats—though codified in another language— the same discourse that the myth proffers in the terms of a narrative. Narration of what happened, a piece of history, the structure of a biography? Yes, but on condition that we remember that the structuring of that piece of biography is similar to the distribution of iron shavings in a magnetic field. The configuration of the iron shavings depends neither on the metallic dust nor on the experimenter's will. It depends neither on the analyst's theoretical model nor on the analysand's biographical events. It is the image of a subjacent reality to which the historical is subordinated: the *mythical structure*. That mythical structure, made manifest by the construction, is universal and ahistorical. It affirms that a paranatural, supernatural order is in standing. It attempts to say the ineffable. It postulates, *on the basis of lack*, the existence of *what it is* (which is because it is not that): the Numinous. Its divine condition is grasped on the basis of the human creature's orphaned state. To be a son or daughter, to have a father. This means the postulation, based on castration, of the existence of a phallus. The phallus of another, an Other to whom I am joined by a filial relation. Therefore, a phallus that is potentially mine. That myth—constructed to give an illusory response to the questions about the origins and the end of life (which is death) and about the meaning of death (hoped to be a rebirth into a new life) and also about sex and the vicissitudes of love and hate—is the very heart of any construction. The heart, but not the skin. This epidermis, all that is apparent and extrinsic with which the mythical structure dresses up for its epiphany, refers to the contingencies of biography and the crossroads of history. Salvaging the historical (reconstruction) is a valid task only if in this process of mnemic recovery and of invention of connections that correlate pieces of history, we can read, as if it were transparent, what is upholding the historical construction: the myth. This means, as Freud teaches us, a truth that is truer than reality. Therefore, why not recognize, without beating around the bush, that it is a mythical construction, inhabiting an eternal present in which historical truth is secondary, though not entirely dispensable, since it is the connective tissue that the mythical requires in order to establish itself and to affirm itself there.

The notion of construction in Freud hardly adheres to the notion of historical fidelity. History can be unfaithful to the facts only if it intends to have meaning. This meaning comes from the universe of things that are nearer than facts. And that in a broad sense determine those facts. Just as they determine dreams. Not only dreams but also biographies are failed attempts to realize wishes. A biography—I quote from Shakespeare—is made of the stuff that dreams are made of. These dreams that are us.

At this point in my text, I feel that I must not continue to elude the urgency of posing some problems relating to historiography. Psychoanalysis belongs (at least in part) to the historical sciences. The importance, doubtless, of the infantile biography and of the cultural medium in which it unfolds. (By the way, if all scientific disciplines imply, to different degrees, a more or less artificial cutout, we must recognize that the cutout that leads to configure this recent cultural object called psychoanalysis is certainly strange. A cutout that runs through, *inter alia*, all the natural sciences, the historical sciences, linguistics and sociology. Psychoanalysis is not only a tributary of these sciences. It also renews, revolutionizes, and impregnates them.)

Historiography: A Two-Way Lane

It is indispensable to differentiate what we call history from the raw material (an unstructured, chaotic mass of things that happened) out of which history is made, structured, constructed, in a process of selection and of linkages, decreed by the historian's mind. The indiscrimination between two concepts that are frequently mixed and confused in the word *history*, that of the *res gestae* and that of the *narratio rerum gestarum* (that is, "the things that happen" and "the things that are narrated"), implies a fallacy. The raw material of the infinite things that happen is not yet history. It would not be so, even if its chaotic registration were possible. History is only the structure that I construct, describe, and communicate. For that construction (verbalized) I use, it is true, raw material that is the things that happen. But these are only an aleatory and dubious, unstructured chronicle of what happened. This registration, on the other hand, is impossible (1) because it can be no more than partial, and its removal from an ideal totality invalidates it; (2) because, far from being faithful, it carries the indelible mark of the instrument used for the register (and this is its original sin); and (3) because what happened is factic, whose meaning (the famous "meaning of history") is impossible to discover unless it is removed from a usually cryptic reality made of elements such as wishes, affects, anxiety, guilt, narcissism, and the drive. In sum, a metaphoric magnetic field to which the factic elements— the iron shavings—are subordinate so that on the basis of that subordination they can acquire a meaning that is not their own but rather borrowed. (What meaning of its own could the white underwear of the Wolf Man's parents have, when the child was 1½, during that nap of fever and sex, if the structuring of his Oedipus complex at age 4 had not enabled him to re-signify what was registered retroactively [*Nachträglichkeit*]? That is, by re-

signifying it, to infuse it with meaning and for that reason to metamorphose it into history, into what we call
history. As the register structured by an intention that
lends it its meaning.)

When Freud, at the beginning of his career, gives
the first definition of *the* psychoanalytic practice, calling
it an attempt to fill in the mnemic lacunae, he introduces,
without mentioning it, the concept of construction. The
notion of construction was born in Freud's mind simultaneously with the notion of interpretation (although at
the beginning of his career as an investigator he believed
that he had given interpretation a higher status). It happens that here, too, nature is horrified by emptiness, and
the destructuring of the symptomatic substitute formation or false connection is inevitably associated with the
structuring of another connection with a supposedly
substituted formation. Which is precisely the one that
the Freudian construction attempts to salvage and proposes. Then what is history? A mere register of the factic,
therefore, it is not. It is, let's say, a structure that I, a
psychoanalyst (meaning a historian), as a structuring
subject, organize with portions of that raw material,
which I select for constructing according to a certain
order, a narrative that says or postulates the *logic of the
facts*. (Oh, the illusion that facts in themselves could be
logical!) I am the one who decides on the criteria of ordering. I respect that raw material in order to use it to
construct one of the infinite combinations possible. I will

take into account the psychological, the economic, the political, the individual, the social, or other criteria. History is that structure pregnant with meaning. *Pregnant from the outside.* Impregnated by a myth. A myth that I, as a historian, choose according to my will, with my convictions (and convenience). A myth that I, as a biographer, intent on looking at reality from my particular psychoanalytic view, discover (after having inoculated it with smuggled goods) in the productions (constructions) of the "facts" that I will later call historical.

Well, let us study that psychoanalytic historical criterion to which we have assigned privileged status. What is it? It is a structure that holds us prisoners, that imposes itself on us, that lives on us, that orders our lives. Unconsciously. It is the myth that . . . we are. It is the truth of our being. Our discourse says that truth in different ways. For example, through our biography. A constructed biography tranfusing the life-giving sap of the myth into the register of the facts that, in their infinite variety and multiplicity, lend themselves to anything.

In sum, history, which is no longer chronological, is myth. To be more precise, a myth constructed (like Evemere) with pieces of the factic registered in life lived. It is the same myth that leads us to dream. How deep Calderon's "Life is dream"! The comparison between life (seen as the facts of waking life) and dream (seen as the hallucinations of sleep) is affirmed by the mythical organization that underlies both products. Formations of the unconscious. Both dreams and waking life. We suddenly understand what waking life is: no less than dream, a motivated construction given meaning by the myth. And that the events that occur are often determined by the mythical (re-)signification they can later take on.

To Freud's "the present repeats the past" let us add the crypto-Freudian (meaning his less explicit thinking) "the past is constructed in the image of something present: the mythical structure. The past copies and repeats the present."

The Interpretation, the Construction, and Their Objectives

We know that the princeps instrument of psychoanalytic therapy is the interpretation. When Freud speaks to us of other processes and other curative mechanisms such as construction, working through, mnemic recovery, verbalization, the transferential relationship, and the anaclitic type of relation that the patient establishes with the therapist, he is referring to processes that are not always absolutely specific and exclusive to psychoanalysis. However, the interpretation is. The interpretation that, for Freud, operates on the transference, attempting (in vain) to dissolve it, acts in a diametrically opposite way to the techniques proposed by the other psychotherapies, which stimulate it, take care of it, and cultivate it in order to derive profit from its condition as the best channel for inoculating orders and suggestions. All the psychotherapies use the transference like the canvas on which the painter—the psychotherapist—applies colors. They proceed *per via del porre*, as Leonardo da Vinci put it. Psychoanalysis, however, is the therapy that, far from fortifying and using the transference, tends rather to destroy it, to stamp it out, meaning to erase the trace of a bridge-image that, like a screen, comes between patient and analyst. Thus, at the end of this operation, the relation between the two will be denuded and a link (relationship, exchange, communication) between those two characters, analyst and patient, without the intermediation of transferred imagoes or of anachronistic, recycled affects, can be attempted. Analysis, as Freud would say, along the lines of Leonardo's paragon, proceeds *per via del levare*—like a sculpture. Interpretation. A process that in encountering a symptom, a dream, a parapraxis, or the transference, just as it occurs live and direct in the crucible of the analytic situation, always operates in the same way and aims at the same goal. What is the objective? To dissolve, to eliminate, or, more precisely, to *destructure*. But we must ask ourselves: destructure what? With this question we place ourselves at the threshold of the Freudian discovery. The answer that dawning psychoanalysis proposes originates in the first steps of the investigation that Freud undertook, and it is categorical and definite. It is the destructuring of the *false connection* between a wish drive and a substitute formation. False connection and substitute formation are two concepts that refer to the same process. This is undoubtedly the basic notion of psychoanalytic psychopathology. I remember having said that if I were ever cornered and forced to say in a few seconds what I consider the Freudian discovery of greatest transcendence for the understanding of human behavior, I believe I would answer: the notion of *substitution*. We live in a universe of substitutions, of substitutable objects. And the core of human behavior lies in that capacity for substitution. One signifier is substituted for another. Because on the human plane life is discourse, the *anthropos* speaks through his or her different manifestations and symptoms and equally in dreams or parapraxes. The acts of our life, syntagmatically combined, are our language. A symptom, for example, is a piece of discourse constructed with its own particular syntaxis (primary process). It can be read, deciphered, translated. Of course, it also happens that symptoms can be studied in the light of a causal relation. That is, they can be taken as effects of a cause or of a constellation of causal factors. However, the great turning point that characterizes the Freudian discovery, in its view of symptoms, is precisely that it turns its back (Freud does it almost without noticing) on the investigation of the causal relation and centers its attention on the investigation of the relation of meaning. Freud does not wonder where the symptoms come from or what agent causes them. Freud, revolutionary that he was, wonders what the symptoms mean, what things they are the signifiers for, what meaning they refer to. Freud, faced with symptoms, wonders whether they have a meaning as a phrase can have a meaning, even when it is mutilated, or as the page of a book when it is full of lacunae and hiatuses. Here, Freud seems to divorce himself from the field of the natural sciences, in which the medicine of his time is proudly inserted and, giving in to an old inclination, turns toward the human sciences, marked by the notion of *intentionality of consciousness.* (Husserl, who by a strange coincidence was also born in 1856, was doubtless not an author perused by Freud. However, how can we avoid seeing again that in the history of ideas people do not create certain currents of thought, but are taken over by them here and there, and are led by them to proffer things, in different contexts and languages, that are marked by an amazing analogy?) Human sciences, marked by meaning, by sense. Faced with the question that Freud himself asks: Do symptoms, like dreams, have or lack a meaning? Freud shows us no hesitation. His answer is Yes, symptoms have a meaning. Symptoms do not present us, as they had until that moment, with a disorganized and chaotic group of manifestations resulting from the destructuring of something previously coherent that has broken (the shattered symphony of a demented musician). All to the contrary, we find a coherent construction with its own grammar and rules of codification. A coherence that always refers to a meaning. *Logic* is operating. The logic that governs the primary process or magic thought. Logic centered on the legitimacy of the most unexpected processes of substitution. Unexpected, absurd substitutions not only of synonyms but of antonyms and paronyms, disconcerting from the viewpoint of Aristotelian logic and its basic principle, the *principle of identity*. (A is A for logic. A can be B, C, etc., for the primary process.) The primary process proclaims the legitimacy of substitution in any piece of discourse. Returning to the thread of our discussion, I will finish the reconstruction of that moment of the Freudian discovery. A mythical moment whose supposed illumination summarizes a process that was actually gradual, advancing in a sequence of partial intuitions and inferences. Freud, identifying with Champollion, conjectured that the apparently absurd discourses of the neurotic symptom or of dreams communicate an arcane and secret meaning to the person who knows how to understand their message. Freud proposed to discover the key for the decodification of the new hieroglyph and achieved it. The morning of July 24, 1895 (the dream of the injection of Irma), was nearly a facsimile of the same miraculous illumination that shook Champollion on September 14, 1822. Champollion ran toward his elder brother, shouting excitedly, *"Je tiens l'affaire!"* [I've got the thing!] and fainted. In the same way, Freud, who was not yet 40, wrote to his chosen "elder brother," Wilhelm Fliess, "Do you suppose that some day a marble tablet will be placed on the house inscribed with these words?—In This House, on July 24th, 1895 the Secret of Dreams was Revealed to Dr. Sigm. Freud." In this way, the manifest signifier covering the latent signifier is set aside, and the latent is recodified and expressed in a different manifest signifier.

(A parenthesis that in a way anticipates one of the theses of this chapter: a current theoretical model proposes a dual interrelation between manifest and latent content, with a two-way bridge that determines the codification of the latent into the manifest and the decodification of the manifest into the latent. I consider this implies a fallacy. In order to dissipate it, I propose another model: the manifest signifier is destructured by the interpretation that undoes the false connection; the latent signifier now needs another signifier to manifest it: this one is constructed so that the latent can be placed into it and expressed by it. Therefore, there is actually a triangular trajectory: from the cryptic manifest of the symptom, which *alludes by eluding*, and is put together via primary process, reaching the latent, palpitating, and concealed heart; and from the latent or what is alluded to, the signified, to a new signifying structure that says it or declares it in another way that we call the primary process. In that new signifying structure we recognize the construction, not according to its 1937 definition but according to a wider and more basic definition. In sum, a double translation. Or, to be more precise, first a deciphering—a path that goes from the manifest of the symptom to the latent meaning—then a translation, a path from the latent meaning to its expression in a piece, a constructed piece, of logical discourse. In other words, one of the definitions of the term *construction* represents nothing more than the translation of a latent content into English. Construction, therefore, of a logical syntagma. I close the parenthesis underscoring that in this context the term *logical construction* refers to a historical definition different from that of 1937. I shall take up the discussion of the latter definition in another section of this chapter.)

Freud investigates and discovers the essence of the psychoanalytic method: the interpretation. Freud is not an unfortunate Etruscologist who limits himself to conjecturing the hypothesis of a hopelessly lost language. His Rosetta stone, his dream of Irma, enables him to discover the key. An obvious key: Colon's egg. The dream or the symptom is a puzzle that must be disassembled into its constituent parts in order to substitute these for others and put together a new, intelligible structure. Freud uses his key time and again. Then, he makes his other discovery: the dream is a realization of wishes. Wishes that one's ego will (dis)inform through substitutes. Which *elude* cogitation of the true wish: *the triumph of repression*. Which *allude* to it: *the failure of repression*.

More than fifteen years afterward, Ferdinand de Saussure, a man from Geneva, posed the problem of human
discourse in terms of a structure whose lines of force
and underlying skeleton result from the integration of
two different procedures: combination and substitution.
The syntagmatic and paradigmatic axes that symbolize
them integrate a model that accounts for the nature and
the dynamics inherent to the structure of language.
When we speak we combine units of discourse into
constructions. Constructions that establish a relation of
bi-univocal correspondence between a signifier and a
signified, permitting logical language, coherent grammar, discourse—in sum, obeying the principle of identity.
Things combine with each other, but each is at all times
equal to itself. This is the Freudian secondary process,
called logical thought. Freud pushed the discovery of
Ferdinand de Saussure, termed the *system* of language,
to its ultimate consequences. Saussure says that in order
to construct the different syntagmas, we sometimes appeal to the mechanism of substitution, which enables us
to preserve a certain combination by using substitutes
within a relatively invariant scheme. Freud, who never
read the master from Geneva and was immersed in the
investigation of another field of phenomena, took this
argument to the extreme and demonstrated that this
substitution can happen against all logic and in flagrant
violation of the Aristotelian principle of identity. A
meaning can be said through countless signifiers. The

relation of a stable bi-univocal correspondence is therefore definitely discarded. A can be said through the mention of B, C, and so on. We may think, without departing too far from the thinking of the first (end-of-the-century) Freud, that A is the *original*. Therefore, B, C, and so on are translations or substitute formations that have connected (illicitly, from the logical viewpoint) with a certain desiderative drive having a certain affect. Therefore, this is a false connection, with a formation that is not the "true one" but only a representation that substitutes for it. Later, Freud discovered that this formation is also a structure in the strictest sense of the word. And he also discovered that it is constructed on the basis of a conflict between mutually opposing elements that integrate, thanks to the ego's synthetic function, into a compromise construction, a *Kompromisbildung*.

After this preamble, I imagine that the reader will have formed a fairly clear idea of what I (and Freud too, I believe) consider the *interpretation* to be. It is viewed as an operation, a discursive activity with a specific function: to undo false connections, to pulverize those compromise structures that we call substitute formations. The interpretation breaks, destroys, destructures, pulls apart, unties, undoes connections that Freud considers and terms false, since they are inadequate, being substitutes for another, more legitimate connection, and being compromise structures in which the wish must necessarily settle accounts with anxiety.

It is clear, then, that *interpretation* and *construction* are not only not synonyms, not interchangeable, but operations that are frankly opposed to each other. While the interpretation destructures, the realization of a construction, as the word says, means structuring and materializing an assembly of separate pieces. The construction integrates, combines, puts together. In sum, it "restitutes" something that replaces the thing destroyed by the interpretation.

It could be thought, in line with Freudian theory, that once resistance is overcome and repression cancelled, the desiderative drive could unite with what (what would it be?) the substitute formation was replacing. However, the ever-recurrent resistance impedes this wished-for union between the desiderative drive and the "original" object that was its aim, proposing another alternative substitute to the ego, if not directly a new edition of the same substitute structure (as in the case of symptoms that persist beyond the interpretation).

On the other hand, to make an analytic construction is to put together a logical structure and offer it to the desiderative drive so that the latter mistakes it for a valid, even viable, substitute formation. Thus, despite its exotic taste to the palate of the unconscious (cooked on slow heat by the secondary process), the desiderative drive will treat it as if it were a new *symptom*. That is, libidinally bound to it. The construction (with the same structure as symptoms) is a product that snuffs out anxiety and satisfies an erotic wish. It derives its value and standing from offering the patient the same possibility for realizing wishes as the symptom. It is, if you wish, an artificial symptom, constructed *ad hoc* by the analyst so that, through sublimation, the patient renounces past stormy loves (symptoms) and couples, with less suffering but with less jouissance, with a more "reasonable" mate (actually, more reasoned and constructed).

After this affirmation, I can finally say, following the tracks of Freudian thought, that a construction is a way of substituting a symptomatic substitute formation with a privileged substitute formation that attempts to say, in a language respectful of the norms of logical thought, that same myth that is the essence of the symptom, the essence of the symptomatic substitute formation.

The Myth Pulls the Strings

I think that without departing too far from the subject I have proposed to discuss in these few pages, it would be a good idea to make explicit my viewpoint on the ultimate reality, whose habitat is the unconscious and which accounts for what is most specific to the human condition. I think that the ultimate reality, the aim of psychoanalytic unveiling, is the myth. A myth truer than reality, if we consider reality the factic, historical, contingent reality through which the myth is expressed. In all human behavior, we can intuit the existence of an ineffable formation for which I find no better term than the word *myth*.

I could have said, as is commonly said, phantasms, unconscious fantasy, latent thought, regressive wish, and so on. I prefer the term *myth* because it refers to a generic, group fact that arises from the intersubjectivity inherent to the human condition. The myth that is expressed in the dreams of every human being, the myth that refers to the universal dreams of today's primitive mankind, the myth that we find when we disembowel the structure of symptoms, of parapraxes, of humor. Now, if a substitute formation is assembled in function of a myth that is transfused to it from another structure or a supposedly true connection, then we can see that the main function of the construction that the analyst proposes to the patient is to give that myth back to the patient, a myth that was orphaned from its support when the symptomatic substitute formation was pulverized. That myth is the main ingredient, the quintessence of a new, logical, and verbalized structure, through which the analyst tries to salvage a truth and offer it to the patient substitutively. "Give me your symptom and I will give you a construction; that says just what your symptom says; that will make you just as happy as your symptom does." This means that the analyst's construction is not the sought-for truth either, but simply a *contingent appara-*

tus that relates to the infantile biography and accounts for the myth that was previously said or spoken by the symptom. In sum, a substitute, verbal, and logical formation constructed by the analyst takes the place of another preverbal and alogical substitute formation defensively structured by the patient.

When we speak of construction, we must refer to the material from which that construction is made. And to the craftsman or constructor. As for the construction material, we have no choice but to recognize its contingent, historical, factic character. Spurious material, therefore, one might think. But not so spurious (Freud would retort) if we bear in mind that when the desiderative drive is displaced onto any substitute formation, it gives it meaning and the value that it carries from its original relation with the substitute formation. In the construction, it is altogether a substitute formation that has been privileged, ennobled, and dignified by the drive that resignifies it when it cathects it.

Six More Postulations on the Construction

First, the construction's main objective is to stimulate the patient to produce more and more new material: confirming, rectifying, mnemic, intellectual, affective material. Second, its structure is symptom-like, implying compromise and substitution. Third, it is different from the symptom proper because it is put together, unlike the symptom, *via the secondary process*. Fourth, it is a libidinal object cathected by the patient, whose therapeutic power derives from that erotic relationship. Fifth, it can be constructed only on the empty lot left by the previous destructive action of the interpretation. Sixth, its appeal to the memory is fallacious: it does not try to dress itself in screen memories; it attempts to view the myth naked.

I would like to go back for a moment to some semantic implications of the term *construction*. In the second line of the fourth paragraph of his article "Constructions in Analysis" (1937 p. 259), Freud offers the reader who prefers it (!) the alternative of saying "reconstruction" instead of "construction." That prefix *re* seems to destroy my thesis that the process of construction aims at a new and ahistoric architecture. That same paragraph reveals the model with which Freud attempts to justify his argument: archeology. I confess that for me, this is one of the texts in which Freud commits a flagrant contradiction of the supposed parallel between psychoanalysis and archeology. Let us reread this page. You may be surprised to observe that Freud underscores, as what is most important, the differences between archeological reconstruction and psychoanalytic construction. The arguments follow one after the other, and everything points to the same conclusion: psychoanalysis has to deal not with dead and mutilated remains but with something alive that evidently (to Freud's mind) determines the special configuration of the construction. If instead of archeology Freud had looked for a metaphoric example in biology, he might have been able to tell us more clearly what he was really thinking: a living organism, mutilated in special historical circumstances (the day, the hour, the place, etc.), attempts the reparative reconstruction of new tissue, independent of those so-called historical circumstances, acting only in function of the atemporal and ahistorical natural laws that govern its biological behavior (or, in our case, its mythical behavior).

Because I have signalled the profound similarity between the symptomatic substitute formations and constructions, which I also consider substitute formations, it is important for me to underscore certain differential characteristics that may tend to make us believe that the construction lies at the very antipodes of symptom formation. Those differential characteristics, enumerated in part above, certainly exist and are as follows:

1. The construction is an artificial product constructed from and by logical thought.
2. It implies a lower quantity of repression and therefore a stricter relation with a supposed founding activity of the false connection.

3. It has a certain coherence and plausibility that yields a certain degree of conviction that is therapeutically useful for the patient (even when it brings up no memories).

4. It is made not by the patient but mainly by the psychoanalyst who has for that moment left aside his or her activity as interpreter.

5. It exercises an important function because by replacing the symptomatic substitute formation and by being cathected (by libidinal displacement), it produces an *artifact*, to which the patient can cling while on the sea of anxiety of the pathological primary process and feel, though shipwrecked, that he or she can let go of his or her symptom because there is an alternative life-vest, one of whose characteristics is that it realizes a sexual wish. (Frequently, the enthusiasm of the erotic transference moves, and is transmuted, to intellectual enthusiasm for the constructions proposed by the analyst.)

Up to now, I have said that two of the main activities through which the psychoanalytic process takes place are the destructuring interpretation and the structuring construction of new formations that replace the substitute formations that have been interpreted and destroyed. I have pointed out that the interpretation is opposite to the construction, just as destructuring is opposed to the ever-restitutive structuring. I have also suggested implicitly that all construction infers a previous destructuring, just as the architecture of any new building infers the bulldozer that knocks down the building that existed on the site before. As I have pointed out, construction for Freud involves organization. That construction is an operation accomplished by the psychoanalyst with the patient's cooperation, conscious or not. That childhood history, especially the elements that can be considered screen memories of the prehistoric period covered over by infantile amnesia, is important. Why? Because although they are a contingent form able to dress up the myth, those "historical" events represent the singularity of each archeological reconstruction. I have said that what is really constructed is a myth and that this myth is the same one underlying the symptom. I have also said that just as every substitute formation is a compromise structure, so too is the construction that the psychoanalyst puts together. It remains for me to make explicit once again that although Freud sometimes presents the construction in the material of a case history as the cause of certain symptoms, it is actually no more than a signifier that tends to patent a certain meaning. I doubt that we can speak simply, as some would like, of causality, and I think that we should follow the elucidation of a relation of signification in which the historical construction and the myth are correlatively signifier and signified.

A Daring but Not Heretical Hypothesis: Transference in Reverse

Wrong-way transference? No. Simply two-way. That is, we must think not only of a re-edition of the past in the here and now but also of a re-edition of the here and now that is punctually repeated in a past whose structure is inspired by a current model.

There is something else I would like to say about the construction. I believe not only that it is important to underscore what has been said up to now about constructions, in the sense that they reflect a mythical reality that forms the internal structure, the skeleton, of symptomatic discourse, but that we would be well advised not to lose sight of construction as one of the vicissitudes of the analytic process.

The Reading of the Individual History and the Simultaneous Unpublished Writing of the Psychoanalytic Adventure

By this I mean that in the moment that the analyst proposes a construction, he or she not only alludes to a piece of past history and to its relation with a re-edition in the here and now (the transference) but also makes current and prospective history. In other words, the construction accounts for (1) a founding myth, (2) its historical costume (infantile biography), and (3) its re-edition in the transference. But the construction also represents the moment in which, in the field of the transference neurosis, the analyst writes something personal, inscribed as an event in the history of the psychoanalytic treatment. Which is another history not yet published. An example will make it clearer. When Freud interprets the symptomatology to the Wolf Man, constructing the model of the primary scene episode, at five o'clock in the afternoon on a summer day when the feverish patient witnesses his parents' coitus, that construction is not only the transcription to a spoken language of what was registered in code in the symptoms of the Wolf Man. Aside from this, something happens there that motivates the writing and reading of past history to form a pretext, a reason, or a starting point for a new history, "the novel of the treatment." I will give you an example. In the fifth canto of his *Inferno*, Dante tells us that Paolo and Francesca, the two unfortunate adulterous lovers, were one day reading the novel of the love between Sir Lancelot and Queen Guinevere. Their reading led them not only to feel moved by the vicissitudes of the protagonists but, carried away by their emotions, to kiss each other. At that moment, the reading of the love story of Lancelot and Guinevere is an episode in their writing of their own love story. They believed they were copying the love of the couple in the book. In reality, the opposite happened to them. On the basis of the current experience of their own love, they re-signified the relationship between Lancelot and Guinevere as being identical to their own love. Past history is re-signified on the basis of present history. Therefore, not only does a present copy the past, but a past is structured in the image of the present. Freud, together with his patient, is experiencing an adventure, the adventure of the psychoanalytic investigation of the Wolf Man's illness. This investigation and its vicissitudes form the novel they write together in the here and now of the analytic situation. And the result of that investigation that delves into the past is inevitably colored by the vicissitudes of the current relationship. Taking this argument to its extreme, we could contribute a new and enriching approach to the Freudian proposal: the analytic construction does not uncover history. It invents it. And this invention functions therapeutically, even when, as Freud reminds us, the patient is unable to recover the memory! I believe all this opens up a new path that has nothing to do with the subject of transference neurosis (which is re-edition), but with the subject of the relationship with the analyst (which is a first edition).

In this sense, I can affirm that during psychoanalytic treatment, we apparently read a history that the patient brings to us, written in its cryptic language, that we must decipher with the patient and read with him or her. But what is actually most important is that we also write the history that we experience together and that we link it to the deciphered history. What does this have to do with the subject of constructions? Answer: what we construct, taking it back into the past, is the secret diary (to give it a concrete name) in which we register the current events of the relation with the patient but conjugate the verbs in the past.

Returning to linguistics, let us go back to the scheme Saussure proposed regarding the construction of language, on the basis of an axis of combinations or syntagmatic axis and an axis of substitution or paradigmatic axis. We can say that the interpretation involves work that is done on the paradigmatic axis, the axis of substitutions. The interpretation means replacing the substitute formation for something that represents the substitute formation, perhaps a bit more precisely. On the other hand, the construction is a process that involves an attempt to combine visual and conjectured elements by way of an operation that consists of linkages, unions, and combinations. That is, it is work done all along the syntagmatic axis. Using linguistic terminology, I would say it this way: the construction is a *syntagma*, while the interpretation is the destructuring of a syntagma resorting to the process of *paradigmatic substitution*. I can't resist the temptation to use an allegory. I know that I abuse metaphors and similes. But could someone please suggest a way, if it exists, of alluding to the essence of things if not through metaphoric language?

It is known that Renaissance painters often had no blank canvasses and therefore painted on those that had a pre-existing painting. Paintings have been discovered, as art critics and historians know, at the moment the outer painting was scraped away. I believe that constructions given in an analysis can sometimes be compared to that second painting, which as we know is no facsimile of the underlying painting but something else. Something else and the same thing. Because for the painter it is a way of repeating the myth that he attempted to say with his first painting. The two paintings don't need to look alike. However, although they are different, they do look like the same myth, of which they are only formally different versions.

It seems the time has arrived to address the question that I formulated above. Who is the constructor? The myth, which speaks from the analyst's mouth. But we must not be blinded by the evidence. The patient also constructs. And sometimes, as Freud says, those constructions are what we call his delusion: a construction in any case! Perhaps the most reasonable answer on the authorship of the construction would be: the authentic author of the construction is the myth, which makes itself heard through the voice of its emissaries—the analyst–patient couple. Integrated in a complementary relation, they evidence a bit of construction by the analyst and another bit of delusion of the patient. (And also, we say *sotto voce*, a bit of the patient's construction and a bit of the analyst's delusion?)

Summing up (by way of synthesis for the reader who has opted not to read the above reflections):

History does not exist until we invent it.

The invention is based on the myth that is each of us.

The myth attempts to place *something* of what transcends it into an anecdotic structure, of which it is merely one version.

That something is the Numinous. It is the affirmation (spoken out of lack): It exists.

The register of what has happened (sometimes faithful to a certain factic reality and sometimes hallucinated in a dream-like way by memory) is simple and complacent raw material from which the myth borrows certain bits.

Historiography is a two-way street: from past to present (repeating the act) and from present to past (copying the meaning).

Interpretation and logical construction are diametrically opposed and indissolubly linked.

Historical construction involves a logical structure and something more: a restitution (following the destruction effected by the interpretation); a symptom-like compromise; a mode and an object of libidinal gratification (by way of sublimation); the use of the register of what has happened as if it were the preconscious day residues of dream work; a disguised *transfusion* of the myth into the very heart of the history.

To interpret is to separate what is artificially and illicitly stuck together.

To construct is to read or formulate something legible.

Psychoanalytic treatment means reading the history (corrected by the interpretation); it means experiencing it in the transference neurosis. But it also means writing a new history. So psychoanalysis is pure mirror? And what about the frame?

2

The Mystery of Time

Mauricio Abadi

Le temps s'en va. Le temps s'en va, Madame,
Las, le temps non, mais nous nous en allons.
[Time passes. Time passes, Madame,
Alas, it's not time, but we who pass.]

Ronsard

Time. We all know—we believe we know—what thing this is. Intuitively. Submerged in it, our existence goes by, without our consciousness that we have been accessories, on the basis of the norms of a certain culture, of a distorted experience in our perception of time. Culture—do you prefer to call it ideology?—decides for us what thing time, its perception or rather its construction, *must* be.

Time, says Shakespeare in a famous line, is the stuff that life is made of. From the inaugural moment when someone plunges us—traumatically (the birth trauma, *Hilflosigkeit*)—into that universe, marked by temporality, until the instant in which our internal clock indicates that the time has come and a decisive strike called by our functions throws us out—with some external help usually—of the flow of the stream that dazzled Heraclitus, and there we are, bathed in time. Someone plunges us in, I have just said. Is it really this? And really, does our exit from the eternal present of intrauterine life and our consequent entry into the temporality of drives and desires represent the expulsion from the earthly Paradise? An expulsion decreed by someone, God, the parents of whom we are born? Or is it rather our *will to be born*—you can read or reread *Renacimiento de Edipo* (*The Rebirth of Oedipus*, Abadi 1960)—that leads us to escape from the Nothingness that held us prisoners? Thus, we can choose to exist accepting death, rather than the nonbeing of entrapment in a hermetic eternity. An eternity that, since it is no more than a continuous present, is foreign to time. Meaning foreign to narration. And therefore to that which the narration serves: "the invention" of meaning. (Perhaps you would prefer to say—more Freudianly—to the recognition of a meaning that pre-exists its discovery. So be it. Do you like it better that way? I don't. I prefer not to renounce to a certain doubt.)

Time. The Greeks fancied it—in the image of humankind—as a God who devoured his children. A god(dess) who enables us, *vellens nolens*, to exist along a segment with an end point in order to reincorporate us and thus return us to Nothingness.

The god Kronos, the symbol of that pedophilic cannibalism, only lightly masked by an orthographic variation (Kronos instead of Chronos), cannot conceal, in his condition as Chronos—Time—the ephemeral beat that throbs in the very heart of life. Kronos, avid to reinternalize the same life he engenders (and which escapes him), devours his own children. Just as Chronos (time) does.

How can we fail to remember at this point what Vernant and Vidal-Naquet (1972) tell us: that among the founding laws of metamorphosis, in which a latent process of culturization culminates, among the laws promoting the burst (birth-delivery) that originated a new and unheard-of coexistence, aside from and above (without ever eliminating) that other legality that reigns in the natural jungle, there is a law? Generally unknown. *It is the law that prohibits us from eating our children.* There are, we know, basically three of these founding laws. However, curiously enough, in all the time since anthropologists first laid the bases of contemporary ethnography, they have mentioned only two: the *prohibition of parricide* and the *prohibition of incest* (interdictions that actually refer to the same thing, which means the forced dependence of the children possessed. Since being a father implies having displaced from the bedroom, meaning killed, the father, in order to take his place. That veto on cohabitation with the mother, in the marriage bed, is the symbol of all the laws that humankind structures in its attempt to preserve the social organization that establishes itself from threatened invasion by natural legality, which stalks the social being from the jungle. Freud would have said from the sea, in his tenacious attempt to recover the land, like the land salvaged by the Dutch, from Nothingness.)

But we close this parenthesis, whose only purpose is to remind me of the scheme of a theory I proposed in other works and that postulates the radical unity of the apparent binomial: incest and parricide. The prohibition of incest is equal to the prohibition of parricide and also equal, therefore, to the dependence of the captured child.

Three—as I said—are the founding laws that preside over our social and cultural organization.

We have already discussed the two that are most mentioned. We must bring up the third. It is none less than the prohibition of eating one's own children (*tekna* is Greek for "offspring"). Creating a new word with two Greek roots, I once termed the practice of eating one's own children (though perhaps ritualized and veiled later) *tecnophagia*. (We may well wonder what would have happened in the development of Freudian thought, and hence in psychoanalysis, if Freud had been more inspired by *The Bacchae* than by *Oedipus Rex*.) This practice derives from an instinct that pursues the survival of the individual more intently than the perpetuation of the species. The law in question, the law that prohibits *tecnophagia*, signals a foundational milestone in the epiphany of culture and in the transmutation of the more primitive hordes into human societies. Ruled by certain laws, more or less systematically groupable in a coherent and global organization of norms (which is culture), humankind tries to subdue the jungle (a jungle reigned over by animal egocentrism, rivalry, envy, jealousy, and greed in their boldest manifestations). Freud has taught us that all these impulses, since the sanctioning of those laws, are subjected to psychic forces—the usual ones, those of the drive—but *now* directed inward. From this moment on, they will be known and recognized as *repressed forces*. Forces that impose the direction of new existential itineraries. *Detouring* or creating the neuroses and their sublimations, or *stopping* at the barrier and *marching in place*. Marching in place means "to move without advancing." It is something like performing *inactive actions*. Inactive actions or movements originating in an impulse and moving outward, ex-motions, *emotions*. Or in other words, ad-fects, *affects* that are set up inside where there might instead have been ex-fects, *effects*—facts expressed outward, toward the world. Has anyone thought—I wonder—(although the Stoics knew it) that *the emotions are actions that, when they meet with a barrier, bounce back inside?* (I am not deliberately speaking of repression. Since repression in psychoanalytic terminology is something else. I am speaking of suppression, Freud's *Unterdruckung*.) Therefore, there are no affects, I believe, unless there is something that opposes them. Have you thought that the affects are effects that could not be? Or that the connate and volitive spheres of old-fashioned psychology are the same as the affective sphere and vice versa? Ideation, emotion, and action are the same thing, different vicissitudes of the same energy. Therefore, what is wished is already happening. This was obvious for Catholic theology, which speaks of the sin of intention. Freud also knew it in the instant in which a sudden illumination enabled him to understand that the desire to re-edit the primal experience of satisfaction appears to be the "practical," "factic" experience of a hallucination. *Ergo*, the expression "identity of perception" is ultimately a different way of expressing what I propose as the identity between the affective sphere (of desire) and the active sphere (of the experience of satisfaction). This means that the *desire* (and the affect associated with it) is the other side of the *action*: the obverse and the reverse.

I now conclude with all these digressions and go straight to the point. *The subject is time.* Or to be more precise, as the title reads, conceptions of the mystery of temporality, which intellectuals, scientists, and philosophers before Freud tried to elucidate in the past. I can perhaps propose some of Freud's ideas for a conception, with a psychoanalytic bias (still incomplete!), of time. Ideas that enable us to delve into the unconscious of the human being who concocted and protagonized them.

Clearly, conceptions of time are the trademark of different cultures. Each culture has its own conception of time. Time may be considered a reality in itself, independent of the things that move in it (the absolutist conception) and also may be thought of as a relation between things, in the order of simultaneity or of sequence (relationist conception). Our conception of time always turns upon a subjacent fantasy, conscious or not: an entity, "continuous, homogenous, and always flowing in the same way" (Ferrater Mora 1965, p. 786). On the one hand, there is the absolutist conception, represented predominantly by Newton and the most fundamentalist Newtonians, and on the other hand, there is the relationist conception held by Leibniz. I pass quickly over the Kantian conception, the notion of time as a *necessary* representation of experience, an *a priori* category of sensibility, a pure concept of understanding in the sense of an intuition. This is a dereification of Newtonian time. In passing, I also mention the Hegelian conception of time as "Spirit" *in its unfolding* (since Spirit in itself is nontemporal or eternal) and time is its unfolding. As in other, more modern conceptions: the temporalism of the romantic philosophies; Dilthey and his historical time; Bergson and the intuition of a "real duration"; Heidegger and his preoccupation with finding a foundation for the notion of Being in temporality; and so on. Until we reach the dazzling culmination (no, I'm not idealizing Freud; I'm only recognizing that he put his finger on it), the psychoanalytic understanding that things and events have meaning only if they are susceptible of narration. That is, of something for which the postulation of a lineal sequence (time) is indispensable—whether mythical or real, no matter. What matters is that without that sequence (or time) there is no narration possible. And without narration there is no *meaning*. Not even a compass with which to find it. And if there is no meaning (I would say, paraphrasing of what Voltaire said of God), we would have to *invent* one (which is, perhaps, what we analysts do?). Without meaning there is nothing but *meaninglessness*, chaos, nothing, Nothingness.

Our admiration for Freud does not stop here. There is more. After having postulated the need of time as sequence, he blows up that sequence, breaking lineality into pieces. But for now we shall take up the thread again before I get lost.

Is it not striking that the philosophy books are lacking in allusions to the revolutionary Freudian conception of time? I think that it must not be simply because Freud failed to elaborate a systematic theory of his conception of temporality (*Freud is valuable especially because he didn't bother to be systematic!*), but because reading him arouses inevitable resistance—for two reasons: (1) because of the reference to the evocation of a traumatic past, buried by infantile amnesia; and (2) because of the reference to anxiety about the passing of time (*tempus fugit*) and about death: the limit where time, the only thing that counts, which is personal and untransferable, seems to stop. Like the notion of *repetition*, which like a broken record turns around certain traumatic facts that seem to stop the temporal flow and that act either as magnets for attraction backward (regression) or as modulators of a flow marked by the "faster" or "slower" velocity of a sequence.

Some conceptions—for example, the river of Heraclitus—speak of the anxiety about what cannot be stopped and held. Others postulate (wishful thinking) that time is nearly like an empty frame in which humans gradually outline the profile of their lives. The latter conception originates in an attempt to deny the passing of time and to eternalize it by immobilizing it.

Other conceptions (or rather, ideologies, wishes, fantasies?)—in Plato, for example—dissociate the flow of time from the immobility of the eternal. Saint Augustine, on the other hand, renounces any definition because he feels that in the very attempt to define time, he loses it. Newton throws him the gauntlet and challenges him: this is Newtonian time. Others place themselves at the edge of its flow, look at it—or try to—from the outside, and settle into some of the varied forms of appetite for eternity such as Buddhism, Zen Buddhism, the mystics. There are those who anticipate it (futurologists) or else reactualize it in the memory (historiographers). Or who accommodate themselves in it like a driver at the wheel who intends to drive it (politicians). But let us look at this and also something more, in detail.

Among the conceptions of time that have in some way surfaced in human consciousness and found some attempt at formulation, more or less scientific or philosophical, in different periods and authors, I will begin by enumerating, first, the *mythical time* of religions. It is a time of *eternity*. It is the time whose meaning is trans-

parent in the word *everness* or in the German *Ewigkeit*. It
is an *atemporal* time. A time equal to itself, immutable
and we could almost say, forcing the meaning of words,
a *temporal space*: a place where things happen. Or it is, if
you like, one of the dimensions of space. It is a time
beyond deterioration and creativity or any progressive
or regressive change. A time whose immutability and
perfection (the perfection of the sphere, we could say,
borrowing a metaphor from the Eleatics) reflect, as if it
were one of its principal attributes, the essential trait of
the Numinous, of Divinity. The time that appears as eternal is nearly the symbol and mirror where humankind
can look and look at itself, intuiting the invisible form
of God.

Opposed to this *entelechia* is a time made of changes,
of mutations, a *time of historical happening* whose transformations are inscribed more in history or in culture
than in natural legality. Although in nature, too, there
are changes, but in a cyclical way, as with the seasons,
the reverse of what happens in historical becoming where
the changes point toward a certain end or denouement,
culmination, final catastrophe, or metahistory. That time,
which I call *the time of change*, is the time of creativity but
also, as Aristotle said, the time of deterioration. It is a
time, conceivable as a static force, not that of the wind,
but rather of stagnant water, that acts on the things that
are inserted into its space and wears them out and also
transmutes them, creating new entities that take the

place of those that disappear. It is time as an agent of change. Of those changes that history is made of. Therefore, it refers to the notion of historical or biographical time. Freud, it goes without saying, is inserted in this conception. It is the time of narration, of the narratable. Because he knew that only in the underground of the narration (not necessarily historical, but rather mythical, somewhat masked as a real, factic, biographical thing) will we encounter the meaning again. The psychoanalyst is, as we know, a truffle dog. I am translating an Italian expression, *cane de tartufi*. Have you ever seen one of these superspecialized canines? They sniff and dig, dig and sniff at the earth until they find the truffle. Just as we—the meaning is the truffle—listen and remove, with *words*, the sod of the conscious material until we come across the precious hidden meaning. I said we remove with words. I didn't say with interpretations. Sometimes, often, these removal words don't interpret. Their function is different. To provoke, to stimulate, to motivate, to irritate, to condition responses. Provoking agents, that's what we are, in our best moments. The interpretation is only *one* of the possible provocations. But this has to do with the subject of time only very indirectly. I mention it here in passing only so that you will (re)read my paper on interpretation. And rethink some of the dogmas that we repeat uncritically without thinking them over. Sometimes, we need only add *credo quia absurdum* (I believe it because it is absurd).

In third place (third? I've lost count) there is a conception of *lineal time*, a time conjectured or imagined as
a lineal trace, an itinerary that is there (as if it were a
highway), which human beings travel from beginning
to end or rather, since it has no end, to the moment they
must interrupt the trip and leave it. Time, the highway,
goes on. It is lineal and infinite time. This lineal time is
perhaps one of the principal forms in which the course
of existence was imagined for centuries, conceived of
as narratable temporality. We can add *finite lineal time*,
a subvariation of this lineal time, time that has an end.
The end that is also the end it aims at: *metahistory*. A
paradisiac state, a mirror image, for the future, of the
mythical Golden Age or of Paradise Lost, where humans
live in radical and absolute atemporality. As before the
Fall and our expulsion into the universe of time. It is the
biblical and Christian conception of time. A time that
begins with the Fall and ends with the Redemption. The
space between fall and redemption is the hard time of
life, which for a psychoanalyst means the punishment
to expiate the guilt of the fall (fall equals birth for me).
As in Dante's Purgatory, expiation has a limit. And redemption initiates a timeless state, the "city of God" for
Saint Augustine or perfect coexistence in a metahistory
for the Marxists.

Another alternative category: a *flowing time*, that of
the *panta rei*. This metaphor suggests not a highway but
a river, and time is the water in the river that flows.

Heraclitus and his thinking (expressed in a [formally apocryphal] saying: "Nobody bathes twice in the same river") accounts for this conception that condemns us to a paradoxical immobility, like Prometheus bound to the flow of time. A time that is made visible to us, I would add, since the water of the river is diaphanous and invisible, by the things it sweeps along: these things are the "others" who in dizzying succession appear and disappear. "*Tout passe, tout casse, tout lasse*" [Everything passes, everything breaks, everything tires]. We add, like the cynic, "*et tout se remplace*" [and everything is replaced]. And the substitute not only *names* the nostalgia of what it was, with no possible return; it also *lies* by saying that nothing happened, that everything is still there.

Cyclical time: "do you remember?" is the well-known conjecture of a circular time, time that is repeated as a cycle, just as the *theory of the eternal return* proposes (Nietzsche among others). The matrix of this fantasy of cyclical time is certainly the cycle of the seasons and the interminable succession of deaths and births.

There is a *Newtonian time*, I said above, or a time in which the temporal dimension seems to be correlated and deduced from the relation between velocity and space. We are now, doubtless, in the august presence of science. However, we know since Freud's contribution that the process of magical thought is primary and that it underlies and buttresses discursive and scientific thinking. This time—a stage on which two giants, infinite space and mythical velocity, confront each other, the latter desiring instantaneousness and ubiquity or the defeat of space—seems like a time of the Formula I, a time that tries to achieve, beyond the sound barrier, the annulment of distance and of separation.

Einsteinian time. Relativized by the curve of space and by a time integrated as a fourth dimension into the traditional family of the three dimensions of space. Regarding this Einsteinian time, I will summarize the idea that Ferrater Mora (1965) offers us. In the Newtonian conception, the nucleus of the problem is that the measurements of the flow of time are "relative" to an absolute time that "flows uniformly, unrelated to anything external" (p. 787). In the theory of relativity,

> time (absolute in Newton) is "relativized" when it becomes entirely a function of a variable system of reference from which all observations and measurements are made. For this reason, there is no "absolute" simultaneity, and an event can be simultaneous in relation to one observer but not to another observer. [p. 788]

God, the privileged and absolute observer of the cosmos and in a way foreign to it as the Creator is to its creature, has died. The theory of relativity strikes down his attribute as a unique referent. A democratic polytheism has dethroned the protagonist of monotheism. Thus, the laws of the universe are the same or equally valid for all observers.

Not to speak of the conception of time in intra-atomic physical processes, which obliges us to reset the question of whether time is continuous or discontinuous, whether granular or irregular. But about this discontinuous time I don't think I can speak. If any of my readers would like to accept the challenge that physics flaunts at psychology, I happily concede you the floor.

Going back to our enumeration, there is a *calendar time* with its yesterday, today, and tomorrow.

There is a *past time*, which is the time of *present memory*.

And a *future time* (of desire and anxiety), which is the time of *present expectation*.

And a *present time*, qualitatively heterogeneous in relation to the past and the future, which paradoxically tends to flee from itself, attracted to two magnets: the preterit and what is to be.

There is also a paradoxical "before time appeared." Before the "Fiat lux" of the Bible. Before the "big bang" of the astronomers. And a *time of death* that is actually the death of time. Of time as life.

There is a *biological time* that investigations of the recent decades have detected in the time it takes children's wounds to heal in comparison to old people's. This scarring is a nearly mathematical indicator of the different biological times pertaining to the different developmental moments of life.

. . . and a *psychological time*, the interminable time of the misencounter and the quasi-orgasmic time of the encounter. Also, the problem of psychological time has been broadly (though incompletely) explored, and Freud made a weighty contribution when he investigated the time a dream lasts objectively compared to the time it lasts for the dreamer, observing the hiatus between the two (just as he drew our attention to the different times in the simultaneous processes of *scenification* [*Darstellung*, display] and in the successive processes of secondary elaboration, both in dream work and in waking life).

The Christian conception of time begins with Saint Augustine: "When they don't ask me I know; when they ask me, I don't know." We would do well to compare this with *dreaming*, for which the same can be said, and remember as an example a very brief and dizzying Chinese fable. Lao Tse dreamed that he was a butterfly, and when he awoke he no longer knew whether he was Lao Tse or a butterfly dreaming that it was Lao Tse. There is a *social time*—for example, the time of appointments, of the opening and closing of banks or offices. A time that society, intent on cultural parameters, encloses dictatorially between parentheses.

. . . and a *quantifiable economic time*, not Newtonian as a relation between space and velocity but as a relation between capital and interest rates. (I might remind you that, apropos of the latter, one of the fathers of the

Church, later canonized, studied the problem from the theological point of view and condemned usury and even the charging of any interest, however small, resorting to an argument related to time (!). He argued that what is paid with bank interest is not capital, property of the lender, which is supposedly returned intact, but the *alienation time* of that property. And since time belongs to God, not to the lender, a human being cannot receive gain for something that belongs to another (and what an Other!).

We must remember finally (isn't a psychoanalyst a historian?) the *time of historiographers*: epochs, periods, generations. And the credible hinges that historians give us for articulating those different moments: 1492, 1789, not to speak of the incredible year 0 of our era, which entered occidental history as the year 1.

And why not speak, finally, of the *life time* or *expectancy* that insurance companies are so interested in?

Lastly, there is a notion of time based on the *time of duration* (which brings us to Henri Bergson). How is duration felt? Could it be experienced as a reassuring permanence in the face of anxiety of change (of death), or as a threatening reality opposed to the wish for change? Duration of the waiting room. A painful waiting room, because it postpones the wished-for moment. And a fearful waiting room, since it draws us close to the moment of the realization of the persecutory threat. The particular inflections that Henri Bergson (Ferrater Mora 1965,

p. 791) gives to the question of the problem of time are, I believe, three:

1. He shows that the structure of our thinking, of our scientific theories and conceptions, of our *episteme* (as Michel Foucault would say), is notably *spatialized*. And that this is our way of eluding recognition of the unavoidable temporalization of life.
2. He shows that *duration* is the basis of time.
3. He shows that the sentiment of temporality is an object of the *intuition*.

There is a word that for us (psychotherapists that we are!) is opposed to duration: it is *urgency*. Urgency begs loudly for duration to end.

In any case, to end this brief review, we must recognize that there are two basic categorizations of time: one is characterized by the before and the after, which are thinkable entities (perhaps myths, perhaps illusory fictions), and the other is the instant, the Now that we experience. That instant, I think, has nothing to do with the time of before and after. It is neither a phantom of the past nor a fantasy of the future. It is experiential, nearly visceral reality. We must not fall into the ingenuous error of considering the present as a hinge that articulates the past and the future. It is instead a feeling, the perception of something ineffable, it is rhythm, life, that attempts to flow, which I then let go of and am left without, without that painful and joyful consciousness of it. Consciousness of my existence. Consciousness that I am alive.

Before going on to the psychoanalytic conception of time, I propose a review and a rethink on some questions. Is time a *quantum* or quantifiable matter? Does it exist *per se* (ingenuous realism as one of the *a priori* categories that, according to the illustrious professor from Königsberg, the human mind orchestrates in the process of apprehending the universe)?

Is time a continuous entity like the water of Heraclitus's river, or is it a discrete entity? Is it infinitely divisible, as Zenon of Elea proposed implicitly with his strange demonstration of Achilles and the tortoise? And as the equally respectable owners of Rolex, Girard Perregaux, explain it?

Well, I shall stop here. The list could be infinite.

No, I want to add something more. There is a time that greatly interests psychologists and sociologists. The *full* time (as full as that of a pieceworker) and *free* time, a basic preoccupation of our civilization: time without use, for which an appropriate use must be found. On the pain of *boredom*. If you look at it intently, against the light, you will infer (I couldn't say see) what is really there, concealed behind the boredom: nonbeing.

We have at last come to the conceptions that psychoanalysis and the psychology associated with it propose to us in a revolutionary way.

1. There is a time of the systems:

a. A time of the preconscious system, with traces groupable as "past," made up of successions, alive in a re-updatable memory file. Re-updatable because of the expectations sustained by the cathexes of our unconscious wishes, and ordered because a principle of reality that substitutes the pleasure principle is in standing.

b. A time of the unconscious system with traces that associate among each other with absolute simultaneity behind the chain that presided over the creation of the traces.

c. A time of the present conscious (a few seconds, according to the latest investigations in the laboratories of experimental psychology), in which preconscious traces make a sudden and ephemeral appearance, pushed up from a metaphoric "underneath" by the traces and wishes of the unconscious system.

2. There is a time resignified *a posteriori* or the Freudian conception of the *Nachtraglichkeit*. It is a nonsequential time, it is said. It would be better to say nonlineal. A time capable of infinite and different structurings, but not at all subordinated to the lineal sequence of time as we conventionally conceive of it. *It is a time in which things are ordered in function of meanings, not of chronological sequence.* Meanings that sometimes coincide with

the moment of the "fact" and more often than not originate in an after (the *a posteriori*) and also (why not?) in a
before (a noncausal but meaningful *a priori*). It is a universe made of correlatable mnemic traces (meaning that
they can acquire meaning) and of drive and desiderative
cathexes that, like a magnet, modify the orientation of
the infinite correlations possible. It is a time of my past
history, which I narrate to myself (what does historical
truth matter?) in order to account for *my present "desire."*

3. Psychoanalysis on the subject of time teaches
us that something relating to repetition is a key to the
understanding of the problem of time. To repeat: What
is that? It means trying to deny the passage of time, to
affirm it in an eternal present, to annul any progression
and regression, to defeat it, that winged messenger of
death. Psychotics know that. Their catatonic immobility, sometimes associated with reiteration, is another
attempt to deny the passage of time, which has thus
stopped being the matrix of hope and has become the
black cloud that presages the storm.

But also the *repeating of transference*, whose latent intention is *not to repeat*(!) but to rectify, *to innovate.* Had
you thought of it? That subject who, in full swing of
his or her transference neurosis, repeats and repeats pat-
terns of behavior and symptoms, does it *in order to stop
repeating.* The intention of the phonograph needle, captured by the groove, is to jump out of the groove. Its
ultimate goal is to free itself from repetition.

4. There is a *time of absence* that *is not* time absent but *painfully present*. And there is a *present time* that is a reiterated insistence on *leaving*. (We reread Saint Augustine, the first candidate for a well-deserved Nobel prize from our "couchopolis.")

5. And there is the *time available* in the little ice cubes of the Freudian *Niederschriften* (inscriptions) that melt and return to their condition as drinking water for the consumer. For this reason, precisely, it is the time of representations or of *presentifications*.

I think it is basic for the construction of a psychoanalytic theory of time to not only think of time, which is life gone by and attempts to perpetuate itself in a presentification (through representations), but also to bear in mind that time means unfiling and updating that filed away meaning by stuffing it with new meanings that come to it from the present, meaning the wish, *Nachträglichkeit*. (I know that I said it a moment ago, but I feel the need to say it again. Isn't it important to understand time as merely an *invented signifier?* Behind which there is no meaning at all?)

Up to now, I have hardly mentioned one dimension of time: the future. A future that has already happened, hidden in the myth that attempts to give our life meaning.

That illusory time, which is the time of the future and of the realization of the wish, is contaminated by the time of anxiety. Thus, our ambivalence toward that time to come.

By introducing the basic notion of the primary process (in opposition to the secondary process), psychoanalysis gives us a new way to understand the time of causality and the devilish dialectics between the time of a presence that leaves and the time of an absence that becomes painfully present.

It has also enabled us to understand that time of nostalgia, riding between the irrecoverable past and the future, recovering obstinately and full of flaws. And that time of the memory and its counterpart, amnesia, which—Freud dixit—is a form of memory.

Summarizing the above (nearly devilishly plagued with contradictions and lack of coherence), and trying to synthesize, I would say, schematically, that a psychoanalytic conception of time would try to capture and imprison that hundred-headed hydra in a net made of formulations like those I suggest below.

1. Seen from a psychoanalytic optic, *that* which we call time, *that* which we think we know so much about and which probably exists no more than a necessary fiction of the mind, appears as a structure in which certain elements, meaning *mnemic traces and wishes*, conjugate and interweave in such a manner that they originate the concept (and fantasy) of temporality.

Warning: given the ungraspable condition of the characteristics of temporality, I will have to resort to attempts at a negative definition (apophatic, as Aristotle would have said): time is *not* something. There is a cer-

tain order, changing according to the experiential moment of each subject, that articulates wishes with mnemic
traces or with the ideas deriving from them, not in order
to register a real order but in order to create *new relations of meaning*. The ordering that uses the concepts of
before and after and during, is based on the construction of certain relations of meaning in which before,
after, and during are *signifiers that allude to other referents*.

We say—in the manifest, for example—"before" in
order to refer to another thing, eventually latent, that
can be "good." Thus, the good, an untemporal concept,
is now designated as "before": the Golden Age, Paradise
Lost, and "all past time was better." Or the concept
"after" is articulated unconsciously—for example, with
death—and appears in a sequential plot that alludes to
punishment due to guilt, a consequence of transgression.
Or the concept "during" attempts to account for the
coexistence of antithetic entities such as delivery and
birth, pleasure and pain, *et similia*.

In summary, for psychoanalytic thought, above all,
time *is not*, time *signifies*. It alludes. Poor Time, you pretend to be God and you're nothing but a signifier. (Ex-
cuse the irreverence of my writing. I want to avoid the
starched scientific terminology whenever it doesn't help
us to understand.) *For that reason, time is continually and
eternally destructured and restructured, so that it can be used
as a privileged signifier of life and of death.* Kronos, time, is
life and death; it is what gives life and what gives death.

2. There is an inescapable theme when we speak of time: the theme of *rhythm*. Cardiac rhythm (remember the ideas of Arnaldo Rascovsky on the origins of the notion of time in the fetus, based on the perception of the mother's heartbeat). From here, the rest of the rhythms. Rhythm of music, of poetry, of dance. Rhythm of love and of sex. Rhythm that presides over the creation of the universe and transmutes Chaos into Cosmos.

3. Death anxiety produced the idea of an infinite time that engenders the concept of *eternity*. I believe, therefore, that there is a filial relation between time and eternity. But this can be detected only in the light of the death anxiety that psychoanalytic delving enables us to discover.

Eternity and time. On the manifest plane, the two concepts confront each other and seem to be mutually exclusive. From the beginnings of philosophical discourse, in ancient Greece, the two titans dispute the ambiguous conceptual territory that corresponds to the notion of temporality: eternity and time. A cross-examination is in order. Plato, witness for the prosecution, makes Aion (Eternity) say, "You, oh Time, do not exist, you are a pure reflection or shadow of me, I am the Archetype that you are reduced to." But—Freud willing— we could make Time say, "You, oh Eternity, do not exist. You are simply an illusory fiction, born of the wish for immortality and, beneath the solemn appearance of an intellectual construction, you conceal the matrix that engendered you: your anxiety in the face of the avalanche of time that devours everything."

Finally, although psychoanalysis is born of a theory in which biographical time is placed in the constellation of causalities (childhood with respect to adulthood, for example), it is notably different from any approach to the *post-hoc, ergo propter hoc*, in two key moments in the evolution of Freudian thought. The first, when he leaves aside the seduction theory and discovers that his "neurotic," as he calls her, is the expression of fantasies (even current ones) that are fantasies activated in the here and now. No longer temporal causality that can be relegated to some punctual time zone of the biographical time of childhood, but always present causality that acts on the basis of the mythical wish that inhabits us and moves us. The second, when the discovery of the *Nachtraglichkeit*, the *a posteriori*, breaks away from any vestige, if there was any, of a unidirectional conception of time. The past can be steamrolled by the waves that crash in from the present—retroactively—and change the meaning that a conventional conception of the temporal sequence would seem to impose. What happened "really" (the meaning) when the Wolf Man was 1½ is determined (not predetermined but *postdetermined*) (!) by what happened to him later, when he was 4. From the horizon of the Oedipus complex, the shadow of the primary scene is projected onto the child age 1½–retrospectively and retroactively.

Speaking of a psychoanalytic conception of living, we must therefore consider and question the problem of temporality in a meaningful correlation. Let us see some of its most notorious and remarkable aspects in the form of nearly apodictical enunciations:

a. Time *does not* go by: trauma and fixation.
b. Time "marks time" as it moves (repetition).
c. Time wishes to flee (elaboration and invention of new symptoms), using, or we might say abusing, the reversibility of psychic processes. Of course, to this applies something of the principle of entropy. I mean that in a closed system, something equivalent to the second principle of thermodynamics occurs, and progress toward psychosis can become irreversible. Unless we move into an open system, toward a therapist who in this way justifies the real meaning of his or her job: that of helping the patient to elaborate nonpathological compromises.

4. Time is irremediably attracted backward (regression) by a past trauma that tugs on it and by anxiety about the future that sets up a dam against any advance of the existential task. It is the "I want to go on being a child."

5. Time that is not in memory (in the mnemic evocation) is in the repetitive behavior of the present that
is always a veiled, allusive *reminiscence*. When we act, we
"represent" our memory.

6. Past time *is* present because of its continuous updating, and because it inhabits the present of the
memory or of the reminiscent symptom. And vice versa,
the present time is past, since it is repeating and therefore always projecting the same image of the traumatic
situation that corresponds to the point of fixation.

7. Time is measured—nearly like a drive—as the relation between the tension of life (joy and trembling) and
the peace of Nirvana.

8. Time was constructed gradually in childhood,
and the present time is somehow a mere mock-up of that
true time. (Is this Freudian affirmation valid only for neurotics? I wonder.)

9. Time in Freud is *waiting*. Expectation of the
waited-for event: death. (This is the Freud of the death
drive and of Nirvana.)

10. Time is the *mythos* that enunciates the meaning
of the wish and, having metamorphosed it into *logos*, has
probably been the work of our magic defense mechanisms against death anxiety.

11. Time is the backdrop against which life occurs.
When nothing happens, then only time, almost chemi-
cally pure, is etched on the horizon. And that contact
with time, without the intermediation of anything mean-

ingful is, I believe, the perception of empty duration that we experience as boredom. Boredom is the detector of the Nothingness that time covers up and masks with diverse fetishes.

12. There are zones of greater and lesser density in time.

13. The course of time of the conscious is not a uniform flow, but jumpy happening.

Each of these thirteen asseverations merits an investigation in itself. But for now, enough is enough!

I like the idea of ending this sketch of an essay on the meaning of temporality in psychoanalysis by bringing to mind the famous paragraph that Saint Augustine, a real psychoanalyst *ante litteram*, dedicates to this subject in his *Confessions*.

What then is time? Who could explain it clearly and briefly? Who can understand it in thought in order to be able to say one word about it? And yet, nothing is more familiar or better known than time in our conversations: and in speaking of it, we know quite well what we are saying or what we are told when speaking of time. But what is time itself? If nobody asks me, I know; but if I want to explain it to someone who asks me, then I do not know. What I do say without hesitation is that I know that if nothing happened there would be no past time; and if nothing were forthcoming, there would be no future time and if nothing existed, there would be no present time. But those two times, past and future, how can they be, if the past is no longer and the future is not yet? As for the present, if it were always such and failed to slip into the past, it would not be time but eternity. Therefore, if time is time only if the present slips toward the past, then how can we say that time IS, if its reason for being resides in no longer being? In reality, when we say that time exists, we mean that it tends to not exist. [1984, p. 438]

Postscriptum: Ah! Just now, when I'm coming to the end, I understand (*insight*, we usually say) that the *real question*, on which these cavilations turn obsessively, is nonbeing. But that is what I wanted to talk about! Not about time. (I wanted to talk about time as an antidote for nonbeing. As a mythical invention of the fiction of "being.") Yes, yes, now I understand where I was aiming, laboriously, since I began to reflect on the subject of temporality. There are two things I seem to intuit: nonbeing, nothingness, emptiness—do you prefer to speak of castration?—on the one hand; and on the other, the postulation, necessary for survival, of time—the mendacious and necessary foundation of a fictitious "being." Now that I have understood it, perhaps I had better throw these pages into the wastebasket. And eventually begin others.

I won't do it. It matters more to me to show the road travelled (on which I recognize myself as if in a merciless photograph), with its hesitations, contradictions, and digressions toward dead-end streets, than to proclaim a final and definite conclusion. Besides, definite until when?

3

The Identikit of Psychic Reality

Mauricio Abadi

Psychic reality? First of all, we must define, as well as possible, the complex and ambiguous concept of reality from the semantic viewpoint.

Reality is, apparently, my surroundings, the circumstances in which I am immersed ("circum" is what surrounds me).

This means something that I attempt, perhaps in vain, to define in function of a hypothetical "myself," which I baptize with the name of "I" (not the ego, an instance of the psyche; the "je" and not the "moi" of the French language).

It is the obliged referent that enables me to define, from that position, the "not-I" in which I am immersed and with which I am sometimes confronted. It is precisely that "not-I" that I will call reality. First question or great objection: Is not the "I" subsumed in that reality and is it not therefore part of it?

Yes, but. . . . The "but" aims at the idea that for me, "I" is part of reality only if (1) it is perceived by the "look," and (2) if there is another of whose look I am the object. "Look" and "other": two key concepts. In effect, reality appears to us and begins to take on a configuration as such to the extent that it is "seen" (*sensu lato*) by the organs of perception of someone who places himself or herself "against" the object (the prefix *ob* speaks clearly of a "not-I" with whom I am confronted).

When speaking of looking, I am postulating that reality presents itself to us as such to the extent that it is perceived by someone who cathects it libidinally. This brings up three problems: (1) the fusion into one semantic unit of two concepts that I later learn to differentiate: reality and appearance; (2) the question of psychic reality that, as we shall see, is often characterized by "not" being the object of a direct and immediate perception; and (3) by the libidinal cathexis of the subject. We see what we look at. We look at what our libido, like a seeing-eye dog, indicates to us. This means that the condition sine qua non of the knowledge of reality is to cathect it (or to have cathected it) with desiderative impulses. The cathexis is the entry way to meaning.

Also, the word *other* introduces us fully into an intuition of reality as the most radical and absolute otherness. A certain prejudiced conception leads me to imagine it and conjecture it as being material (primitively, reality is what is touched, smelled, or tasted) and as being objectifiable. Which assumes that it is a referent "common" to the other people I live with (do you see it too? Then it is true and not a hallucination of mine. It is real, a part of reality). As we see, what counts is the testimony of other persons who comfort me with their solidarity in the idea that that is real. Or that it simply is. (Parmenides dixit! If it is real, it is, and if it is, it is real.)

Within this reality, intuitively conceived as a universe (or perhaps better yet, a "pluriverse"?) of things (since even linguistics suggests the pertinence and belonging of the word *things* through the relation of etymological filiation between the word *realitas* and its progenitor *res,* or "thing" in Latin), we can describe entities with specific differences.

This reality is abusively referred to sometimes as a presumed synonym of truth (Parmenides, Hegel); as for its constitution, I suggest aspects relating to what is spatial (the *res extensa* of Descartes) and what is temporal. The latter engendered by a nearly ineffable feeling (read Saint Augustine and his definition of time) of continuity, due in part to the will to be and to remain and, in part, to the need to construct the scaffolding for a feeling of personal identity. Within this reality, I can recognize different realities that are categorizable by different adjectivations referring to them.

One of these is the reality of psychic facts. This reality, perceived intuitively from the start and forever after, is not, however, the object of a perception but rather of a construction and an interpretation of what has been constructed, illusorily termed *perceived reality.*

The reality of psychic facts configures a special reality that psychoanalysis distinguishes and differentiates from other realities, calling it *psychic reality.* This psychic reality, as psychoanalysis conceives of it, is a reality that I can perceive, evoke mnemically, know, recognize, approach, or leave, but it is especially a reality that is not only combinatory but also constructed on the basis of substitutions. A reality, therefore, that is not only syntagmatic (although syntagmae have the dream-like quality of structures only loosely strung together) but also and mainly paradigmatic. This means that it is a complex reality that I construct with different elements. This reality can be only if it already has been, in psychoanalytic terms, cathected. Meaning invested, charged with certain impulses, drives, and wishes.

This cathectization is a condition sine qua non—I reiterate—for psychic reality to acquire a meaning. Meaning is also a specific element of psychic reality, unlike the other material reality, which I can imagine as lacking meaning and simply being the object of a perception, and perhaps eventually a construction of the different elements perceived with the aim of inventing a meaning for them. However, this psychic reality absolutely requires the condition that we call signification or meaning. But this signification requires having previously been invested with affects mainly in the order of the drive and its derivatives, desire and anxiety.

What we call signification is a condition that arises from the peculiar and specific relation between two things: on the one hand, an ideational referent, and on the other, a dynamic component that gives it life.

Therefore, the main feature of this psychic reality is not that it designates elements of a reality eventually deprived of meaning, but rather that it establishes a relation to create meaning according to the type of relation the subject establishes with what is constructed on the basis of perception.

That psychic reality (psychic in function of signification!) may sometimes undergo the process of repression, become nonconscious and configure a group of facts characterized not only by their "unconsciousization" but also by the legislation of their functioning, which is not effected by the so-called secondary process or logical thought but by the government, so to speak, of alogical thought or the primary process.

We know that the key to this primary process, this new legislation that governs the mental functioning of that zone of the unconscious, is the process of substitution that can also be described more Freudianly as the displacement of the cathexes from one mental representation to another.

This unconscious psychic reality, like the conscious one, is conflictive, and the conflict cathected by the impulses is inevitably a conflict of forces. In order to avoid the explosion of this time bomb or conflict, the ego invents compromise formations, which are a compromise not only between desire and prohibition, between superego and id, but also between secondary process and primary process. This means that these compromise formations are governed, as if in an intermediate zone between conscious and unconscious, by a legislation and an executive power that is something like a coalition government that sometimes brings together the legislation of the secondary process with the legislation of the primary process in a way that is not consistent with logic. The compromise formations cohabit this borderline or marginal zone between primary process and secondary process. Therefore, all behavior contains variable proportions of the elements of these two realities, the unconscious and consciousness.

It is true that certain realities such as the dream processes are predominantly tributaries of the primary process. And other realities, like the logical reasoning of a mathematician who attempts to demonstrate a geometric theorem, are tributaries of logical thought or the secondary process. But most of the processes that we call human behavior in daily life are evidently a set of compromise formations or compromises that are created and incubated in that frontier zone between the unconscious and consciousness, between the primary process and the secondary process, or, equally, between the drive wish and internalized social prohibition.

When we speak of psychic reality, we often make the mistake of thinking that it is a reality that can be described as internal; it is internal perhaps only in the sense that it is from the skin inward, but it is external with respect to the ego, which resorts to different mechanisms for relating to it. Therefore, I think that we must leave aside those misleading terms that suggest an opposition between internal reality and external reality. It seems equally uninteresting to speak in terms of a presumed opposition between psychic and material reality.

Another point I consider very important is that everything connected with psychic reality presumes the capacity for distinguishing between the truth or the knowledge and recognition of a certain reality on the one hand and meaning or the relation that we can establish between different aspects of reality on the other.

This means that the relation of significance or meaning pertains not only to psychic reality but also to history, to mythology, to the imaginary, to the symbolic, to the project, and to memories, which are not simply memories of events but are interrelated by a meaning.

A great theme is the subject of the manipulations of psychic reality that Freud studied; reality can variously be known, recognized, repressed, denied, disavowed, repudiated, and substituted. (The most evident aim of these mechanisms, from the viewpoint of the conscious, is that they become unconscious, although what is most important is that they adopt modes of behavior linked to the secondary process.)

And finally, I shall leave for another series of reflections a great theme that has no legitimate place in the area of psychic reality: the lie.

Psychic reality can be characterized as follows:

1. It is the same as conscious reality (see Freud 1900).

2. It is "towed away" (this is what we call repression). Some other maneuvers are probably added to repression.

3. It is unconscious.

4. It is governed by the primary process.

5. It is governed by the pleasure principle.

6. Its language is governed especially by the process of substitution of the signifiers (the paradigmatic predominates over the syntagmatic).

7. It is governed by the symbolic equation by which the sign neither denotes nor connotes the signified but rather is the signified.

8. It is the object of dissembled returns (offshoots) of the repressed.

Postscriptum

I shall add a couple of reflections on the etymology of certain words, which are particularly illustrative of the subjacent psychological plot. I will begin with the relation between the concepts of reality and of truth.

Truth (*verum*) is etymologically what deserves to be believed. Thus, it is related to the word *wera,* which in the Slavic region means "faith." This root can also be corroborated in the Celtic and Germanic areas.

Therefore, just the reverse of what is erroneously thought, what is true is not believed because it supposedly witnesses reality, but because the belief of a stronger group has been imposed, even by force: then it must be the truth.

Once more, the protagonist of all the semantic power of the word continues to be the subject who backs the value of what is true in a linguistic term with the credit given by his or her faith.

Conclusion: the true reality is the one we believe in. But are there no false realities? Apparently there are. They are the ones in which I do not believe and that do not merit my faith. (Here again, I lapse into the perennial error: that of presuming that there are objects that merit faith; when in reality it is precisely because I grant them a certain credit that they become true.)

But if there are false realities, do they deserve the name of reality? Or is it that reality (we take it for granted that it is true) is the only truth? If it is so, it is a kind of tautology. Unless we invert the terms of the equation and say, with Hegel, that the only truth is reality. Which also refers to a kind of tautology.

What is true is that there are many realities. And that there are different types of faith. Therefore, there are many truths, although they contradict each other.

Finally, I want to register a reflection on the Greek words that signify exactly that. Truth and reality refer to the same morpheme: *a-letheia*. Etymologically, "unforgetting." Therefore, the idea of the recovery of something that has been lost for consciousness is present. Lost does not mean erased, since it can be recovered. Freud's brilliant contribution is having suggested the term *repression*, since this concept refers preferably to crossing out, which means to write over, covering up the former, as has happened to the palimpsests. Thus, the truth is what was in some way known and was later— deliberately or not—exiled from consciousness (the Freudian unconscious), if we wish to subscribe to a spatial conception of the mind. However, if we opt for another vision of the mind, we can speak of repression as a temporary suspension of the effects of an idea. Which assumes that the idea in question is not only an inscription but also an energetic charge or cathexis. Then, reality is only what is desired by me. That cathexis is what guarantees the signification. Suddenly, we realize that in our discourse we have slid from a concept of reality and truth toward something more basic, which is meaning or signification. What matters is not that something is or is not (true) but that it has a meaning for me in function of an affective cathexis that guarantees it, subtends it, and converts it into an object of my faith.

Descartes, help me! Can it be thus: I desire; therefore, I believe? I believe and the truth illuminates me? I see the truth and know reality? I know reality and in order to manipulate it as I wish, meaning according to my desires, I invent a language, that of the primary process, which enables me to move around comfortably in this new medium that I call reality? But it happens that when I try to go from what is known and desired to action, my surroundings place limits on me and begin to prune that language until it has become adequate for acting on these surroundings; the secondary process is thus born from this series of limitations. It seems that what we call logical thought assumes previous surgery on the corpus of the primary process.

Finally, in reference to Freud's term *Wirklichkeit,* I would say that because of its connection with work, it points to the idea of doing, and therefore to the idea that you are what you do: that is your reality.

4

Evoked Reality

Mauricio Abadi and Susan Hale Rogers

When we speak of memory on the basis of our long-past learning in school psychology textbooks, we recognize four stages of the mnemic process:

1. the perception of reality or the accumulation of nervous excitations formed from certain stimuli originating in the surroundings of what Freud calls the "not-I" and from what is habitually known as reality

2. the stocking or storage of those perceptions that have recorded what in neurology we usually call engrams, which correspond to the inscription, to say it metaphorically, of the different senso-perceptions that the stimuli of reality have awakened in us on the level of memory

3. the evocation of these engrams at a certain moment

4. recognition, meaning that not only do certain engrams flow out of I don't know what unknown region of the mind into consciousness, and I am almost tempted to say "to the surface of consciousness," but these engrams are also put through a sort of sieve that excludes some and retains others as the true and valid ones. This process is the one that we

commonly call recognition, thanks to which our memory functions.

Obviously, these four stages are neither developmentally nor logically concatenated in such a way that we could easily ascend from one step to the other, but constitute a complex structure that we are trying to classify into four stages or moments only for didactic purposes. For example, the relation between senso-perception and the engraving of engrams is obviously very close, but the distance between the latter and the process of storage is greater, not to speak of the immensity separating the process of storage from that of evocation and recognition.

These notions are certainly important and basic, and although they have certain imperfections, I see no advantage in discarding them; I believe it would be better to construct new conceptualizations on this somehow previous structure I have just described.

These new conceptualizations relate to Freud and the contributions of psychoanalysis. On the one hand, we have a basic concept that is "forgetting." Forgetting is apparently the symmetrical counterpart of memory. However, it assumes the existence of a process by which and through which forgetting is produced. It is hardly a merely passive fact, especially on the basis of Freudian investigation; it is instead an active, deliberate, and intentional process.

When Freud speaks of forgetting, he naturally invokes the concept of repression that enables him to create the notion of unconscious, which contains, so to speak, all the forgotten memories that can be evoked under certain conditions, when the resistance or repression lets them pass, as well as their substitutes, masked in some way, evoked when repression allows them to surface under that guise. But it seems to me that for better understanding of this Freudian conception, we cannot simply point out, on the one hand, that the process of forgetting is such a structured process that we can even say that one of the functions of memory is to forget; without forgetting, we might not be able to remember anything, since everything would be pure and immediate evocation of all the memories. On the other hand, we have a second notion that Freud introduces: the two key concepts of repression and the unconscious. But I think that for psychoanalysts today this seems insufficient. We must add something.

I believe that we must make a very important differentiation between crossing out and erasing. I think that the Freudian thesis is that nothing is erased and everything is crossed out. This is evidently the thesis that I consider closest to reality. At the same time, I think that erasing exists only under certain conditions—for example, in psychopathological processes with demential neurological lesions. But I do coincide with Freud that the crossing out or superposition of inscriptions conceals the original inscription, and that they are multiple in the manner of palimpsests or the pictures the painter has done over another painting. This is not only possible; I think that it is universal. I take it as far as to say that all the memories we have are most assuredly the result of neo-inscriptions or the crossing out of previous, hidden memories. I say this by linking it with what Freud called screen memories. In the line of the thesis I am proposing, all memories are screen memories and we have no original memories of anything at all.

In addition, we should question the meaning of this postulation of an original inscription etched onto a tabula rasa. This possibly does not exist, so that if we begin to remove the series of paintings that were done on our metaphoric painting, if we were to remove the second one, the original would supposedly appear. However, that original painting may be something that is given, already structured by biology and genetics.

The other concept that interests psychoanalysts about memory is the concept of evocation, together with recognition. Psychoanalysts think that this process presupposes a cancellation of the repression or the lifting of a repression as is said, and that since this lifting is always relatively incomplete and never total, it impedes the emergence of the memory in its original condition, allowing only the surfacing of the memory once it has been deformed by the crossing out that has been applied to it. Freud maintains that this crossing out has two basic conditions: on the one hand, it is deliberate and intentional, not at all coincidental; and on the other hand, it is intimately connected to the subject's biography. Not just any signifier can be used for a certain signified, but only those signifiers that are given prerogative by the subject's biography, especially the childhood biography.

The other important point is that by creating a metaphorically spatial medium, called the unconscious, psychoanalysts apparently solve the problem of localizing where these engrams are stored; but we are actually avoiding the question, since we still haven't explained what physioneurological entity corresponds to the thing that Freud called unconscious.

Finally, we must discuss an important aspect of evocation and recognition. I believe that they are a fallacy originating in our desire not to lose contact with reality; there is no such evocation or recognition, but something else that we could call, in psychoanalytic language, interpretation of reality; in less psychoanalytic language, we could call it the deconstruction of reality at one moment, and at another, its reconstruction into new significant structures that allude only to what has been deconstructed.

Lastly, it is important to bear in mind that one aspect of the reality evoked by interpretation has been unfairly accentuated in Freudian theory: the purely intellective aspect of the interpretation. I consider that this reconstruction of the different fragments of deconstructed reality is actually done in function of affects, cathexes, or, to use an older term, wishes. It is on the basis of current wishes that we construct that past reality which we label "memory of an event," although in reality it is not a memory of an event but the invention of an event with material that springs from the past which we use and structure following an architectural design dictated by the libido, by desire, and by fantasy.

Finally, there is another aspect of memory: the question of where it originates or what the psychological intentionality of memory is. It is evident that memory is something that can be understood only in the context of the working through of mourning. I shall explain.

In our contact with reality, in the course of life, we are continually losing contact with the stimuli that produce an impact in us. Those stimuli can be present or absent. In every moment, there is a moment when they are present, but the present mommy suddenly leaves the room, and there is something called absence. The great mistake of classical psychology consisted in believing that there is a present mommy and that when she leaves there is nothing. However, today we know that there is something very important that is called "the absent mother." This absent mother produces pain, anxiety, depression, feelings related to the loss of what the child had. This must be recovered somehow. How is this recovery processed? Through the memory that is therefore an instrument in the service of recovery in the process of working through the mourning for a lost object. Then, the mommy has the label, the present category of absent mother, just as present as, or even more present than, the real mother who was present. This absent mother is inscribed and localized and lives in or inhabits the place we call our memory. She is there not as something stored passively but as a living entity that goes on living and continually evolves and whose age corresponds to each instant of the present moment. This means that when a mother corresponding to the age of 4 is evoked at age 24, her characteristics pertain to the desires of the 24-year-old subject. For this reason, we cannot speak in terms of recognition of the mother she was when the subject was 4.

In addition, the memory that was useful for working through the mourning is the creator—and this is the most important function—of a new reality. I believe that this is the most important concept, because we have been subjected for centuries to a psychological conception according to which memory offered us a duplication or a photocopy of reality. Actually, we now understand that memory creates a new reality and that this new reality is the reality where, ultimately, we are living for something that Heidegger defined: language is man's habitat. We live in the reality of the representatives of reality that we have lost which constitute memory.

This memory can be the object of an eventual description, as inevitably fragmentary as in a poem, a painting, or a sculpture, or more so in a film. But it can also be the object of a construction in which the syntagmatic predominates over the paradigmatic, and this predominance of the syntagmatic over the paradigmatic necessarily involves a lineal sequence that corresponds to what we call the narrative. Therefore, it is a reality that is basically tellable or narratable, which means that it corresponds not at all to the real events that occurred but to a reconstruction. Therefore, when we speak of memory, we must inevitably refer to the way in which memory is manifested, which is through a narrative-type sequence in which the lineal, the temporal, the sequential, and the syntagmatic predominate. We will take up the other extremely important reality, the nucleus of the psychoanalytic process, which is narrative reality, in the next chapter. Not before adding that, intuitively, artists and poets have understood this aspect of memory as an instrument for the working through of mourning. An example is Marcel Proust's writing of his search for time lost. In general, the central idea is that a loss leaves a hollow.

This concept is basic because in speaking of a lost object, it was believed that what was left was only an absence. The super-presence of a hole or a hollow, left as if impressed in plasticine when the object goes away and is lost, was unknown. What is left is something extremely important: the trace. This trace is present and weighs much more heavily than the object we lost. Why does it carry more weight? Because we can fill it in not only with the lost object, if we eventually have the opportunity of recovering it, but with anything else. In this way, memory gives birth to all the imaginary and the world of fantasy.

An important fact, related to this hollow that we fill up and tend to fill, which is what is left when an object has been lost, is the theme that originates in the image called *trompe l'oeil*. The *trompe l'oeil* is a reality that we could perhaps call virtual, as is any reality that belongs to the imaginary and to fantasy.

Perhaps the best way of understanding this idea is to compare it with the idea of historical reality. Historical reality says, "Napoleon lost his last battle at Waterloo." And we can also believe the books written on the basis of historical investigation in the form of historical fiction, in which a virtual reality is postulated: that Napoleon won the Battle of Waterloo.

All this is nonetheless reality and is perhaps more real than the defeat at Waterloo because it is linked to the present wish that is the true constructing agent of our memory of a supposed past. I want to add, on the subject of virtual reality, that on my television program, "Conversing with Mauricio Abadi," I have recently introduced a variation entitled "Who are you, Mr. . . . Shakespeare, Heidegger, Spinoza, and so on." The dialogue takes place between an individual who is dead and has supposedly been resuscitated especially to talk to me and another person in contemporary Buenos Aires. This dialogue, a virtual dialogue, has meaning because the questions that I can ask Shakespeare, for example, are products of my present wish and not of my fictitious insertion into the reality of end-of-the-seventeenth-century London.

5

The Fragmentation of Reality

Mauricio Abadi and Susan Hale Rogers

The mechanism that classical psychology proposes for the description of the process of memory has a basic flaw that is so important that if we overlook it, we cannot possibly understand the real mnemic process.

Classical psychology proposes a scheme whereby

1. each reception of stimuli excites the nervous system and, consequently, the psychic apparatus as well (since the latter depends on the former)
2. those excitations are stored
3. they can be evoked
4. they can be recognized and differentiated from others that might have been evoked simultaneously.

What this scheme lacks is everything relating to the deconstruction of the stimuli that are continually being engraved and stored and also, of course, the evocation afterward in the stage of reconstruction. Thanks to psychoanalysis, investigators have finally been able to detect these deficiencies.

In effect, the mnemic process must be understood today in the light of what we know or believe we know. On the one hand, a quantity of stimuli acts on the senses and on sensorial perception or the organs specific to senso-perception and effect something that we could call a register. They register not the stimuli but the physiological configurations that enter the sensory apparatus. For didactic purposes, it seems useful to establish a metaphoric correlation with what happens in a computer. When the stimulus of the keys we press produces a certain effect, certain characters are registered on the hard disk of the computer.

Let's go on to the second step. At the very moment that those engrams, as they are called in neurology, enter, they are immediately deconstructed or destructured or fragmented according to the mode of functioning of the neurological system. Therefore, what is stored in the memory is never the object just as it was perceived and interpreted, but signals that in themselves have no meaning whatsoever.

At some time, the need to evoke a memory occurs. The evocation must necessarily go through a process of reconstruction on the basis of the fragments of the structure that was formerly deconstructed.

The final point is the one that refers to that reconstruction. Reconstruction follows the initial model not as if to copy it but in function of orders deriving from the current desire or wish.

Therefore, what we believe we remember is what we want to think at that moment; what there is from the past is only the material we use to construct configurations, which we call memories, and whose construction is motivated by the raw material of what happened in the past and by a new architecture that structures them in a different way that tallies with the present wish. By this, we are also saying that all memory of the past is a project of the future.

What psychoanalysis has contributed to the understanding of the process of memory is in my opinion the ensemble of two mechanisms whose absence caused a great deficiency in the understanding of memory as viewed by classical psychology. Those two mechanisms are deconstruction and reconstruction.

The consequence of this contribution is that we now realize that what we remember is never a facsimile of what happened. Memory betrays us, it has been said, and the reason for this betrayal is that memory is there not simply to restitute the past but to restitute it in conditions that correspond to the present wish.

This means that memory is intimately connected to the whole process of the imaginary. This also means that memory cannot be understood if it is isolated from the field of the structure of desire.

Finally, this way of functioning generates a personal mythology. Mythology originates in the wish that things past might be otherwise.

This mythology is what determines the individual's behavior, meaning that no individual today is ever the continuation or prolongation of his or her past or the consequence or the effect of his or her past; instead, people continually construct their own biography on the basis of a mythology born of their wishes. This biography is certainly no historical reality; it can be mythified *a posteriori*; it then becomes a mythical reality that every subject tries, through his or her actions in life, to transform into historical reality.

The Psychopathology of Memory

Memory has certain failings, but psychoanalysis has taught us to distrust what is authentically faulty in them and has shown us that these defects are intentional and therefore represent a success. One of us gave a seminar at one time entitled "Faults and Other Successes," meaning precisely that the parapraxes of memory, for example, are facts that by no means represent a failing in the mnemic process, but rather a success and an achievement because what had been proposed was achieved.

What was the purpose? Simply a reconstruction of the mnemic fragments according to a present wish, as we have been saying in other chapters.

What are the most frequently observed psychopathological manifestations of the memory? We can list some of these: forgetting, cryptomnesia, amnesias, the dysmnesias, the paramnesias, and certain defects that are highly specific because they occur in one or another of the different moments or stages of the mnemic process.

For example, there may be a defect of the memory that manifests itself from the first moment, the moment when the sensory apparatus receives the stimuli and the excitations that these stimuli produce. At that moment, a deliberate fault may already intervene; therefore it ultimately constitutes an achievement of the mechanism of the process of incorporation of stimuli, probably what Freud called *Verwerfung*. It seems evident that this concept is intimately related to the concept of foreclosure created by Lacan. This particular concept of foreclosure alludes to a fault in the memory, a fault in the sense that I have just explained, by which the stimulus that has entered by way of the sensory apparatus is in a sense "spit out" in order to avoid its storage.

Another moment in which the mnemic process may be faulty is the stage of storage. The orthodox Freudian view on this point is too extremist or extreme to be acceptable. Freud seems to imply, to say, or to think that no engram is ever lost or forgotten in the sense of erasure. It is doubtful that this is true. We know of certain pathologies of the mnemic process in which some memories are not even kept in storage in any area of the mind. Freud concentrated his studies on repressed memories, but we must say once again what we have been saying in other parts of this book: for us the repressed or unconscious memories that can be evoked—through interpretation—are memories that have been subjected never to a process of erasure but rather to a process of crossing out. An erased memory is not the same as a crossed-out memory, because the crossed-out memory is not cancelled out but simply covered up by an inscription that is applied on top of it; when it is scraped away, the memory previously crossed out can be found. Therefore, a palimpsest or a painting from the workshop of a Renaissance painter on which a surface can be scratched in order to rediscover something that had previously been written or painted is not the same as when we rewind a cassette and dictate something onto it: the former surface is erased. This is a concept in psychoanalysis fundamental for the understanding of memory.

A third moment is evocation or recall, and here it is quite clear that the phenomena that appear are connected to all the vicissitudes of reconstruction. Of these vicissitudes we can mention amnesia or total forgetting, hypomnesia or partial forgetting or confusion of memories, and hypermnesia, which sometimes leads to the recall of certain moments with excessive clarity, memories illuminated as if by a stroke of lightning. This is a process perhaps intimately related to what is experienced in moments of schizophrenic depersonalization, in which a certain memory takes on life, color, and clarity, and stands out much more distinctly than the other moments. This is because that moment has acquired an important meaning; this brings to mind another Freudian discovery: significations can often be detected because they are marked by a change in the form of what is remembered. This means that if one wishes not to remember a murder, one can replace it with the memory of a natural death; however, that unnatural death will be recalled, or hallucinated in a dream, as a natural death, with the singularity that it is too clear or is seen in colors. Thus, through this formal aspect, it is alluding to the repressed meaning of the murder. (See also the concept of vivid memories that Freud mentions in "Screen Memories" (1899) and other articles.)

The problem of the hypermnesias is particularly interesting and has intrigued scientists for some time, especially when they find cases about which a kind of mythology has been created; these cases are persons who in special states of mind are able to speak languages that they never learned in childhood. It is doubtful that they didn't learn these languages; they have probably heard (or overheard) the words they utter in these states in their family circle in childhood.

We have discussed the paramnesias, which include all the distortions of memory.

Next are the cryptomnesias, memories in which the subject evokes something but thinks it comes from reality rather than from memory. For example, one can write a poem and not realize that one is repeating a poem read in childhood; what the writer believes is an original creation is a memory that has lost the notion that it is a memory.

Finally, there are the screen memories that Freud investigated deeply, one of the most important concepts of psychoanalysis because these are memories that serve to conceal and, at the same time, to say things the subject wants neither to silence nor to speak of openly. They are memories that despite their translation in English as screen memories might be better termed *allusive memories* or *artificial constructions*; here, fantasy has worked on the memories so that the subject can evoke them and at the same time avoid the traumatic impact of a direct confrontation with them.

Memories of traumatic situations have an important feature. They are pathologically fixated and fail to adapt to the laws of memory that imply deconstruction and reconstruction, but instead remain stuck there, like a hard cyst or baseboard that is not easily modified. Fighting against this type of memory, as if trying to damage or destroy it by tooth and nail, the subject repeats it in dreams in a vain attempt to elaborate it, digest it, and eliminate it.

On the subject of memories of traumatic situations, it must be remembered that Freud pointed out something essential: their close connection with the repetition compulsion and, for the Freud of the 1920s, with protomasochism and the death drive.

One important aspect of memory is often forgotten, as if it were considered foreign to the mnemic process, and yet it is the very basis of the entire psychoanalytic theory. This idea is that everything is remembered or evoked, if not through memory, then through the body and the psychosomatic illnesses, often a memory expressed in body language.

With respect to this, it would be interesting to bear in mind that body language is more primitive than the language of the mind, that the language of memory is a symbolic language in which an event, instead of being evoked as in body language in an immediate and direct way or nearly a facsimile, is evoked through a symbol that refers to it.

Finally, the importance of vivid memories is—and we may conjecture that this is their prime unconscious intention—that they become the nucleus and heart of certain personal myths.

One subject that we must bear in mind is what Freud called the process of secondary elaboration, which ultimately belongs to the conscious or preconscious mind. This means that when we wish to remember, we must fix the memories to certain fasteners relating to the categories in standing during waking life, which is the time when we remember, and to the categories of time, space, the notion of causality, and so on. This is important because we must understand that the difficulty of remembering dreams is due not only to what Freud says, to their expression of something that we deliberately wish to ignore—also a very important truth—but to something else that is also a result of one of Freud's contributions: his discovery of the functioning of the unconscious, according to the laws of the primary process.

The laws of the primary process usually tell us meanings in a continuous way. We run the risk of losing them if we fail to fasten them onto certain fasteners or enclose them in certain structures like logical structure or the categories of time and space or the principle of causality. For this reason, when we wake up we don't remember our dreams, though when we are awake and an event occurs, we can narrate it in great detail. This is because during waking life what happens is remembered, since we hook it up to what we could call "settings," "structures," or "organizers" that relate to the logic of the secondary process. This is why Freud speaks of secondary elaboration as the moment in which the dreamer can group together the dream images and, in so doing, join them not in a disordered and chaotic way but according to a certain ordering principle provided by logical thought or the secondary process.

It seems useful at this point to explain more clearly why changes in the formal aspect of the mnemic process express deep meanings concerning events.

A patient said good-bye to his father one night just at the moment when the father was taking off his pants and carefully folding them. At the time, that memory didn't seem to be especially important. However, a few days later the patient left on a trip, and while he was away, he received the news that his father had died. Among the memories that came to mind, the memory of his father carefully folding his trousers after having taken them off stood out as a vivid and very precise memory. Naturally, the precision referred to the meaning of the connection with the last moment, the last fare-well, and also to other meanings attached *a posteriori*. For example, carefully folding the trousers might mean an obsessional character trait or else a testament, since something was being given up in an orderly way. This brings up another point. Secondary elaboration is not limited simply to putting a memory into order; other supernumerary meanings are usually added in the course of time, meanings originally lacking in the same memory.

This explains why, in the course of a psychoanalytic treatment, facts gradually change in the memory; memory is machinery that is fully active, constructing non-stop memories in the present, which are wishes that point to the future, but which carry a label, attached by the machinery, that reads "memories of the past," although they have little relation with the past.

Reality as a Narratable Sequence

Perhaps the key to understanding the intimate mechanism of the psychoanalytic process consists in understanding that everything in human consciousness tends
toward a lineal, syntagmatic construction, also carbon-
copied from the mode of the temporal sequence in
which we live out our lives. This means that something
has meaning or is signified only when it can be constructed narratively. The mere perception and eventual
description of an object says nothing. It is orphaned of
meaning. The meaning arises, for example, in a psychoanalytic treatment when the patient can transform what
she or he feels synchronically into the diachronic reality of something that happened, and that kept happening over time, and is therefore susceptible of being told
or narrated.

Reality as narration is perhaps the most basic element of reality that interests us as psychoanalysts; we call
it *the meaning*. There is no meaning without narratable
reality.

One key question that we must ask is: What is
psychoanalysis? Is it deconstruction of reality—as its
very name, "analysis," seems to indicate—construction of reality, or, even ingenuously, reconstruction of
reality?

The answer, I believe at this point in our knowledge, is clear. Analysis is a process of induction by means of certain stimuli; although there are different kinds, all of them are working toward something that is called the affect or, more technically, the cathexis; these stimuli induce the patient to take fragments and to construct a memory. We must not commit the naïveté of thinking that it is reconstruction. It never can be, except in the cases Freud mentions at the beginning of his investigation into the traumatic neuroses. But even in these cases, we must be suspicious. The memories the patient constructs with or without the help of the psychoanalyst, and with or without the assistance of an interpretation, are the narratable reality that gives a new meaning to the raw material of the past because it cathects that material with wishes drawn from the present. Therefore, psychoanalysis is not deconstruction, because we know that what we carry inside is all deconstructed. There is no reconstruction because what was will never again be. It is construction of a new reality about which it would be better not to discuss whether it is true or until we define quite clearly what we mean by truth; however, we can say that this new reality is valid because it has a use. It is useful for reconstructing the identity of the person in the sense of being something that goes on throughout an entire existence; it is useful for helping a person who is ill to choose to get better or to get well, and it is also useful for thinking.

Ideological Reality

Evidently, we are confronted by one of the manifestations of guilt feelings or conscience, what Freud called the superego. When what we remember is painful because it engenders remorse, we have to justify it, and ideology is an attempt to justify things in order to be able to feel that they are acceptable.

6

The New Creation of
An Old Reality:
The Presence of the Past

Mauricio Abadi

My exposition will be divided into three parts. In the first part I will attempt to define the realms in which the transferential process takes place. I shall also offer a synopsis of the Freudian theory on transference. In the second part, I shall discuss a controversial question relating to one aspect of transference, which is in urgent need of elucidation. In the third part, I shall present my own hypothesis on that hotly debated and polemic aspect and offer my solution to the problem. I start with just a few lines of introduction.

Two Who Are Four

The process Sigmund Freud discovered, and baptized with the term *Uebertragung* (or to express it in an idiom of Latin origin, "transference"), is one of the fundamental discoveries of psychoanalytic research. We know that Freud discovered the ever-present transference only after it had expressed itself to him through one of its effects: resistance. We also know that it is a phenomenon, or rather a process discovered within the context of the psychoanalytic relationship whose existence could go unnoticed not so much because it was not evident, but far more because of the therapist's resistances (as happened to Dr. Josef Breuer with the memorable case of Anna O.). It can, in fact, be verified in any psychotherapy—and, to say it once and for all, in any human relationship.

By this I mean that transference is a relationship. A somewhat different relationship from the one you could candidly suppose exists between a subject and his or her circumstantial partner. It exists insofar as a dual relation between subject and partner is impossible. What really exists is something different: beyond the field of conscious phenomena, any relationship between two is a relationship between four. To simplify things, and only for didactic purposes (leaving countertransference aside), let us say that it is a relationship between three. It happens that the subject (for example, during the course of a psychotherapy, the patient) has to deal not only with the person he or she is circumstantially talking to (who could be called the therapist, or perhaps the real external object). This would make things so easy if only it were possible! The subject also has to deal, in a condensed and confused way, with a part of himself or herself, with an internal and imaginary object that, unawares, he or she fictitiously externalizes, projecting onto that more or less compliant screen that is the "other" person. An "other" who because of this new structure of the relationship has lost something of his or her "otherness" to become a duplicate of the subject's "self," a duplication in which the subject does not recognize himself or herself; there was good reason for his or her attempt to externalize it, which is to say, not to accept it as his or her own. A duplicate in which the other (the therapist) does not recognize himself either, but which he or she shall have to govern during the cure. A duplicate unknown to and for both, but present, alive, and determining the course of the relation. An entity that will attempt to appear as being similar to the therapist so as to hide its secret identity, more than just a likeness, with the patient. Finally, an entity that is not really either of them, but a third that enables us to understand the apparently dual relationship as a really trinitarian one. A relation of three in which it shall be unavoidable to settle accounts with that third, or else misunderstand the whole meaning of the relation. This transferred third, transported from one person (and by one person) toward or onto another person who, not really having much to do with it, will have to carry it along anyway. Thus is the relationship between analyzed and analyst. (The third eludes Freud's observation in Dora's case.) Such is the relation between patient and therapist. The barrier that separates us is also a road that connects us, so long as we pay the toll demanded from us to go through him. *All gnosis is diagnosis.* The genius of Freud illuminates the word *diagnostic* with a new light and salvages its hidden meaning. To go through the barrier-bridge, with all the consequences associated with this journey. Meaning the difficulties in communication or that problem (so acute today) of lack of communication, to which human beings seem condemned. Not only because of their condition as islands frustrated in their calling to be peninsulas, but basically because what joins us—the third—is what separates us. This means the difficulties due to the distortion suffered by the meaning which, due to the refraction in a heterogeneous medium (the internal object), makes misunderstanding the core of every human relation (I love you, because I love someone else!). This means difficulty in setting apart. That invisible third, thrown out by one (the subject) and rejected by the other (the object on which it has been transferred), is a third one, disavowed by both, that becomes invisible insofar as one does not want to see it. He will take his revenge, becoming the Punch-and-Judy man who manipulates the relationship between you and me. Suddenly it becomes dazzlingly clear that every relationship is a relationship between a constructed protagonist and antagonist. They are not what they seem to be; they are not elements coming forward from a supposedly solid and unquestionable reality, but rather constructions, artifices, illusions. Entities that acquire new meaning because of memories, wishes, fears. This relation of a subject with what we are now almost tempted to call "himself" (but we know, thanks to Freud, that this "himself" is ultimately an other corresponding to the experiences of the subject's childhood biography) would merely be a dual and internal relation if the externalization and its fusion with, confusion with, and attribution to an embodied other did not transform it into a devilish relation with an other, the mirror of myself, and a "myself" that is attributed to an other. So then, this relation can be expressed thanks to the catalyzing action of a person who at the same time serves as a projection screen for the inner characters that make up the patient's ego through identifications. The relation suddenly unveils itself to us as no longer dual but triadic. However, this relation is evident as triadic only after having been analyzed and its hidden structure exposed. This triangulation determines the style of the relation and sets limits to certain aspects of the patient's behavior. It is a relation in which what is transferred onto the screen provided by the other covers the eyes of the transferring subject so that he or she is unable to see the true face of the object he or she is using as a screen. This way the object becomes un-known. Later on, eventually, it is re-known, if not as real at least in its specific and characteristic condition.

I. What Is Transference?

My purpose for the first part of this demonstration of my thesis is to draw a rough sketch of what we in a usual and Freudian way call transference. Let us begin by saying that the word *transference* comes from two Latin words, *trans* and *ferre*. It therefore means nothing more than transportation. What is transported? And where, when, what for, and how? The first part is dedicated to trying to answer these questions in a lucid and synthetic way. So as to restrict ourselves to a didactic methodology, I shall use a rule known to English-speaking journalists: The formula of the five *w*'s and one *h*. A mnemotechnic formula that helps one remember six key words: *Who, What, Where, When,* and *Why* (to these five we will add a sixth, *What for*, which indicates the intentionality and therefore the meaning of transferential behavior). Finally, the *h*, standing for *How*, crowns our description of the phenomenon in question.

Let us start with *Who*. Who is transferring? Who is the active agent of this transportation? Three different answers appear in the course of Freud's research, all three of them valid, though they do indicate different contexts. I will now mention them according to their chronological order of appearance.

A first answer is every human being. Every human being, in his or her relation with the addressee (the addressee that in philosophy, in opposition to the subjectum, is called the objectum, or the object), is the active agent of a transportation. The subject of this task, which consists of producing the transportation to and from, is, in the universe of substitution we live in, the human being. Insofar as we are agents of a process of substitution that is the basis of both *Uebertragung* (transference) and *Verschiebung* (shifting). Is transferring not a mechanism closely related to shifting (*Verschiebung*) insofar as both are a way of operating with substitutions?

Second answer: specifically concerning the context of a psychotherapeutic situation, we would say: every patient. Or even better, all those taking part in the psychotherapeutic situation (therefore, also the therapist: this is the substance of what we call countertransference).

Third answer, restricting ourselves even further this time to the specific context of the psychoanalytic situation: every analysand (and every psychoanalyst).

These three answers can be condensed into a fourth, the following: "someone capable of substitutions." I had already hinted at it before; the capability to make substitutions and the act of doing so are the most important facts of human life in the cultural universe that it develops. Human beings are defined, to my understanding, as those capable of substituting one thing for another, one figure for another. Transference, therefore, is also substitution; it is also displacing or shifting affects from one object to another object that replaces it.

Surely at some time we will have asked ourselves why Freud called this process transference and not, as perhaps might have seemed more logical, substitution. Since what is meant after all is a substitution (when, for example, the father figure is substituted by that of the psy-

choanalyst, therapist, or teacher). Freud possibly wanted
to underline the fact that he continued to be Dr. Sigmund Freud, that nobody substituted for him or was
substituted by him. His figure was simply "covered"
(taken as a projection screen) by another that only de-
luded the patient, leading him to overlook the screen's
(Freud's) personal characteristics.

Second question: What is transferred? If we exam-
ine the evolution of the concept of transference histori-
cally, we will see that history shows us the following trajectory. Freud noticed, though not immediately, that his
patients developed a kind of affection or sentimental
relationship toward him that in the beginning did not
strike him as unusual (perhaps—why not?—because of the
natural narcissism of every human being due to which
it might only seem natural to become an object of love
for someone who establishes a rapport with him or her).
Later on, because of his capacity for self-examination and
self-criticism, Freud started to suspect that if his patients
loved him so much, it was because in some previous time
in their lives, more precisely during infancy, they had
developed this kind of affection toward some important
figure in their life, an affect that was now reenacted
toward the figure of the doctor. So we can point out
that Freud's first formulation of what transference is
and what is transferred during the process was his recognition not of the primordial but of the transferred,
imported, secondary, re-edited nature of feelings that

were really intended for the person who initially awoke them. Falling in love becomes logical from the moment the absurd fact, transference, is recognized. This would lead Freud, years later, to the completion of his first discovery: not only is transference responsible for the analysand's and the patient's love, but every love comes from a transference.

Almost simultaneously Freud discovered that not only is a feeling transferred: sometimes that feeling can be positive, a bond of love that causes a wish to come closer, but it can also be negative, a bond of hate or rejection.

Freud called the relations based on the feeling of love positive transference and called those based on the feeling of hate or fear negative transference. Within the positive transference he realized that two notably different forms of transference exist: erotic transference and friendly transference. Though both are forms of positive transference, it cannot be denied that concerning resistance, erotic transference, the negative element that appears during the treatment (because it increases resistance), is a positive affect with negative consequences for the treatment. Who feels like talking of love, especially if it is conflictive and creates guilt, while the short circuit of acting seems more attractive? Acting that by eluding verbalization, remembering, telling, and understanding helps to avoid a clash with the head of Medusa of guilt and castration, and to substitute it for a Priapus (metaphorically speaking) based on endless repetition. On the other hand, the other positive transference, the friendly transference, adequately worked with by the psychoanalyst, can favor a reduction of resistance and aid the establishing and blooming of cooperation, something in the nature of the therapeutic alliance of North American psychoanalysts.

Immediately after this first answer—what is transferred are affects—Freud discovers a second answer almost simultaneously. What is transferred, he tells us, is not only affect but, among these affects, mainly wishes and their permanent companion, anxiety. The wishes thus signified are unconscious for the subject; they are infantile because of their regressive origin and usually linked to libido, the psychological sexual energy. Those desires spring from an original experience of satisfaction, which they unsuccessfully try to repeat.

Then Freud offers us a third answer. He says that the person who transfers certain affects onto the therapist does so because he or she has transferred a certain imago to which his or her libido is fixed. Clearly this third answer offers a new connotation. It is not a matter of emphasizing the affects that the actual analyst awakens when, for example, the father figure is remade upon him. What happens is that the affects the analyst awakens now are not due to his being loved as someone else (the father in this case) was loved then, but due to the fact that the father is still being loved and that his mental representation has been transferred onto the analyst. Once more I want to insist here on the etymological meaning. Representation etymologically means the same as becoming present. This should help us to understand that the mental representation is always constructed out of an absence. It is because the satisfying object has left that I refill the void it left behind by representing it, making it present once again with something that somehow substitutes it. It substitutes it insofar as it hints at it and evokes it. That something I call a mental representation is not a thing I manipulate. It is a process of presentification that makes the past become present, suppresses the absence, magically and delusively making a vanishing presence exist.

Let us also say that the above-mentioned mental representations have acquired a life of their own. They are not pictures I have, but ghosts that have me. Ghosts from childhood. Regression. This means that transference concerns infantile affects, and this is usually a characteristic that helps us to recognize the transferential nature of falling in love. A regressive representation is an infantile representation because regression leads back to childhood. Actually, the previous sentence deserves some completing, almost a correction. Really, when we say that during a regression infantile situations are experienced again, we are saying something that, because it is incomplete, may induce us to misunderstanding. It is not a question of returning to infantile situations, as if magically erasing the experience of having gone through more mature and perhaps adult situations. It is about going back to what is infantile, re-signifying it, giving it new meaning, from the perspective of later experiences. Therefore, regression to infancy is never mere recovery of what has been experienced in the past, but a kind of collage or composition in which the infantile is intimately mixed or connected with aspects that have to do with the subject's later evolution. These aspects, when taken back into infancy, give it a new meaning (*Nachträglichkeit*).

Continuing with the history of the evolution of the concept of transference, we recognize a fourth moment. A fourth answer. If just now we said that what is transferred are the imagoes of objects to which our infantile affects are tied, we are now in a position to ratify what we said, using a new formulation. What we say is that beyond the representation of objects, what is transferred is a whole relational package, if you will allow me to express it in these terms. To say it in a different way, what is transferred are not images but relations. Or to say it in still another way, during the process of transference two persons are fundamentally changed by this process: the patient, who transfers onto himself the image of the child he or she has been and of the relation he or she had, and then there is the "other" person, the addressee on whom the patient transfers the image of, let us say, the father. One is almost tempted to say that there is a double transference. In other words, what is transferred is a whole relationship including both its protagonists, and not only the image of an internal object onto an external object (the therapist).

Finally, there is a fifth stage during which Freud arrives at a formula that to me seems to be the last and conclusive stage in the evolution of his concept of transference. This fifth moment corresponds to the year 1913 and to a fundamental work in the evolution of his ideas: *On Narcissism: An Introduction.* The answer that Freud seems to suggest about transference certainly does lead to the concept of projection, not to the projection of the internalized image of an external object but of part of the ego. Here we start to understand that Freud foresees that the ego is built on the basis of mental representations that have become cores of the ego's identifications. And what is transferred is that analyzed other, now my ego, but also my ego that was once the other. If what is projected in transference are parts of the ego, then in the therapist we can see a part of the subject that is dissociated and placed into a relation that ends up being a relation of one part of the ego with another externalized part of that same structure.

We have given five answers to the question "What is transferred?" We have said that affects, desires, mental representations, interpersonal representations, and parts of the ego are transferred.

Let us now continue with the third question, "Where?"—meaning where to: where does the transferred go? The answer is: toward another, onto another, on another. If we put it this way, the answer confronts us with two problems. The first problem is to find out who the other is. (Let us clearly understand that we now mean the screen, the recipient, the assigned object that is burdened with the projection: the analyst, the therapist, the "you" toward whom my ego is going.) The second problem is a consequence of the grammatical preposition we would use: to, toward, on, onto. Let us first see the problem of the other. Who is he? Let us remember that one of Freud's fundamental discoveries is that of biological helplessness, the *Hilflosigkeit* that produces the experience of defenselessness. In the situation of *Hilflosigkeit*, that defenselessness that makes us lean against someone so as to avoid the anxiety of feeling helpless, seeking protection and a guarantee for our survival (even at the cost of injuring our narcissism), what is established is a bond of dependency that is both tranquilizing and frightening. That dependency implies search for support. To say it in modern psychoanalytic terms, the search for an anaclitic relation. The object of this anaclitic relation will be invested with imagoes, affects, and parts of the ego that will transform it into the recipient and addressee of a narcissistic relation, from which we infer that without an anaclitic or supporting object, there is no possibility for that narcissistic relation that we call transference. So then, this transference involves the coupling of a projected, altered, "othered" narcissistic object with an object that I shall try to make mine because it is an other. What appears here is the symmetrical counterpart of what Freud called narcissism. What results is a relation with someone who is not a part of myself, but someone who, precisely because he is not me, can protect me; this is why narcissism and an anaclitic relation are symmetrical opposites. Now we can better understand that narcissism is a desperate attempt to disavow that anguishing and painful dependency, an attempt to hide away in one's own fortress and tell oneself, I am all there is, I can provide for whatever I need, I am the king, or, as Freud says, His Majesty the Baby.

At the beginning, and for some time, the child will be able to deceive itself about its dependency on others, that is to say, on what has been called its anaclitic relation. The child might, in case the other works in harmonious consonance with his or her own desires, buy the illusion that there is no such other. But at some time, the other will prove to be what he or she is: a solid, compact reality that does not always tally with the subject's desires. A reality that can only be surrendered to and recognized as foreign to the subject and to his or her desires. At that moment the child will have to accept that reality, deal with it, and eventually negotiate with the other. But we know, and Freud teaches us this, the child will do so, cheating in some ways. One of those ways to cheat is transference. It is as if in transferring the child told the other: "It's all right, I recognize you as some-

one different (to me)," but at the same time that this
recognition and acceptance seemingly take place, the
other person is being invaded, colonized, penetrated,
infiltrated by parts of the subject's own ego. The other
is, from this moment onward, transformed by the child
into something like a mirror's reflected image of himself or herself. The child will pretend that he or she ac-
cepts that this is some other one, but retaining his or
her internal certainty that ultimately it is still himself or
herself. This is the process we call transference, and now
we understand where it is that narcissism goes. Precisely
to the place where the transferential process is being
structured.

We know that we could almost describe the psychoanalytic process by saying that it consists in achieving that
the patient may at some time recognize that the other is
another and not a part of himself or herself. This is precisely what a psychoanalytic interpretation consists of.
As Freud says, this is what makes the difference between
psychoanalysis and all the other psychotherapies. With
the other psychotherapies the patient is left with the
belief that the other, the doctor, the psychoanalyst, is
nothing but an image of the patient. Who is the analyst
for the patient? The patient. Source, origin, and meaning of what we might call the *psychotherapeutic misunderstanding*, which, during the course of the psychoanalytic
process, the interpretation tries to dissolve. On the other
hand, this misunderstanding can be used as a means to

exert a specific influence over the patient's behavior, as indeed some psychotherapies do. Inversely, in psychoanalysis, the end is to dissolve that transference and to manage for reality to become otherness. To achieve that, the patient comes to know that he or she is dependent and to know that he or she will not be saved if he or she denies the existence of this dependency, but that he or she grows and develops into a subject still dependent, in an adult rather than an infantile way. Being aware of his or her dependency. In other words, what we call a mature and (in)dependent subject.

The second problem we came across when facing the question of "where?" concerned the grammatical preposition. It might seem that the question is quite irrelevant. Whether we say one transfers on, onto, in, into, over, or toward is for me quite an important matter, because it conveys an idea about the sometimes unconscious fantasy every psychoanalytic theorization rests upon when it tries to imagine the process of transference. It is important to know, for example, that Freud would have preferred to say one transfers "over" (*über*, the prefix of *Uebertragung*), perhaps to try and preserve his own identity and avoid the danger of the image projected onto him, like a cinematographic film, being confused with himself. Others will prefer to say "in," especially some analysts of the English school, who consider the partner to be a trunk or recipient of parts of the ego, which are left to and put into him or her. However it might be, I think that the problem of the grammatical preposition, which tries to account for where that which is transferred is inserted, is an unresolved and not a negligible problem. (I leave aside more recent developments concerning the discussion of skin and of the value of the interpersonal relation between the baby and its mother through the skin, just as I leave aside the discussion of the skin as the limit, the cellular membrane so to speak, where a large part of the psychological metabolism of object relations takes place.)

The fourth question is when the transference takes place. Here, too, I feel tempted to give four answers.

The first, and surely the most important, is: always, during the day, at night, anytime.

Second answer: during any psychotherapy, as well as in any doctor–patient relation.

Third answer: in the psychoanalytic treatment (here again I make a difference, as Freud did, between psychoanalysis and other psychotherapies), because as we know, during psychoanalytic treatment, transference is not only used to induce a therapeutic change (called cure) but also interpreted, elucidated, verbalized, translated into the terms of the secondary process.

Fourth answer: mainly during regressive states. This means the more regression, the more transference. This probably explains the deep transference produced during psychoanalytic treatments, because in these a bigger regression is deliberately induced. This is achieved using certain aspects of the psychoanalytic setting, which place the patient in such an unequal position in relation to the analyst that the consequence is a regressive process.

Finally, we have arrived at the fifth question: Why? We are going to divide this question into two. One is Why? and the other one is What for? Let us remember that psychoanalysis is fundamentally a scientific discipline that tries to salvage the meaning of a given behavior, rather than finding out its cause. Yet we must recognize that at least in the beginning, deeply influenced by his medical training, Freud directed his efforts more toward clearing up of causal relations than toward viewing relations of meaning. Now, if setting aside the answer that considers causality, we search for the "what for" of transference, which means the relations of meanings, we will hit upon the following answers: transference takes place in order to build a relation, to build a bridge toward the other. This statement is daring enough for me to feel obliged to offer the reader some explanation. Do I by chance, supposedly basing myself on Freud, think that one cannot have a relation without transference and that our only way of relating is by means of an intermediate link represented by the image transferred onto an addressee? Of course that is what I think. I am not very sure that my point of view is shared by all the other researchers, but my understanding is that in a way we are islands, and that to connect with each other and hold a certain bond, we must build a bridge that comes forward from within ourselves, like an amoeba's pseudopodia. Transference is that bridge built between subject and partner. It is a paradox: my way of connecting with you and getting to know you is by ascribing to you what actually is mine. All these ideas would lead us to a new theory of knowledge based on psychoanalysis. I would simply put it this way: one makes a transference in order to know the other person, because it is the only way to gain access to the other person and establish communication. We communicate because we are united by what is transferred. It is that communication, that double transference that goes from subject to object and back, that ensures a common ground (communion), which permits us to know the other through ourselves.

The second answer to "what for?" transference is perhaps (and this is how contradictory we human beings are) opposed to the one I have just given. If the answer I have just given is that one transfers in order to get to know the other person, the second answer I now propose is: to unknow the other person. Looking toward the other person is what Freud would have called the epistemophilic drive, the wish to know, the research of reality (with the purpose of controlling it). But, especially since Freud's study of narcissism in 1913, we also know that the child tries, in every possible way, to deny the existence of the other insofar as it is an other, and will accept that other only insofar as he or she is someone His/Her Majesty the Baby can commission with something by his or her own

Almighty will. Thus, transferring, covering the real object with a transferred object, is an attempt to save the narcissistic delusion and to unknow the other person, who is then not accepted as the reality one depends upon. We could add that, confronting transference, the subject transfers, and that this transference is equivalent to one of the ego's defense mechanisms. He transfers to compromise, to make an agreement. As we know, the notion of compromise is one of the pillars of psychoanalytic theory. Although that compromise is conscious (these are the so-called formations of the unconscious: symptoms, dreams, jokes, and transferences), it is an artificial structure elaborated by the ego, which, at the cost of a partial renunciation, integrates the opposing and conflicting elements into a structure that substitutes and overcomes the underlying conflict. But if every dream or symptom is a compromise, we must admit that transference, being a compromise, is also a symptom and a "dreaming awake."

As for the "why?" that asks about the causes, the answer simply leads us toward the repetition compulsion.

We have arrived at the last question about transference: How does one transfer? In which way, or by which psychological mechanisms? One way of answering this would be to recall a particularly apt word, used by Freud, and that word is *projection.* How then does one transfer? Well, projecting. We know that projection is a beautiful expression because it is clear, and it immediately flourished in the psychological circles of our contemporary world. Not only in the stricter sense in which it is used by the psychoanalyst. Today, psychologists, even those resisting psychoanalysis, speak of projections. I do not at all believe that we should quit using such a useful word, especially when we use it to speak about the process of transference. But I do consider it important to point out that we should never lose sight of the fact that it is a metaphor. Actually, nobody really projects. There is only, as classical philosophy would have had it, an attribution by which someone is the screen to which something is attributed. To say to project onto him or her seems to be a way of using the allegory of cinema, which must have been very present in Freud's mind. To this we can associate that when we speak of a projection of one object upon another object, we presuppose a more concrete psychology than the one William James proposed. The fundamental parameter of the psychologies prior to Freud, the parameter of the continuous flow of time, or of the flow of conscience in time, was opposed by Freudian psychology or the idea of a structure. Before Freud, psychology was a science that, like music, developed in the temporal parameter, whereas with Freud, psychology became a discipline that, like painting, is unfolded in the dimensions of a virtual space.

When trying to answer the question of how this transference is made, I would like to suggest an answer that a specific rereading of Freud induced in me. Transference takes place in two different moments, the moments Freud usually speaks about in his writings on neurosis and psychosis. The first moment is that of the destructuring of something that could be the symptom, while the second moment is that of the restructuring (or structuring of something new) that we call transference, which substitutes the destructured symptom. Concerning psychosis, Freud says more or less the same in 1924. A psychotic symptom—for example, a delusion—is constructed by going through a first stage of loss of reality, which is the process of falling apart or destructuring, and a second stage of restitution. Well, what I am saying here is that every transference is equivalent to the production of a restitution, and that therefore a previous stage is involved in every transference, a moment that often goes by without notice, such as the moment of loss of reality, of destructuring a given relational bond. I believe it is important to consider this and we often omit studying this first stage when we are studying transference. Perhaps this stage, whose existence is particularly not obvious, is very brief.

Finally, I would like to suggest something about transference that I consider particularly important. It is the following: what is transferred is always something nonexistent. That is, the object being transferred is, if we would rather call it this way, the phallus. Or, in other words, it is omnipotence, completeness, immortality. The analyst who becomes the object of a transference is the addressee of something the patient hands over with-

out ever having held it himself; the analyst gives something he never had, while the patient, hurt by the *Hilflö-
sigkeit*, hurt by his experience of feeling unprotected and
considering his impotence, his castration, and his unavoidable decline, in a desperate attempt to keep up the
narcissistic fantasy of completeness and immortality,
does something (I would almost dare to call it a trick)
that could be expressed in the following way: "Yes, it's
true reality seems to prove that omnipotence and the
phallus are not mine, that just as Buddha discovered in
a moment of clarity at which he arrived by renouncing
his narcissism, I exist only as a mortal, incomplete, mutilated, declining being." But the patient in transference
would add something like "The fact that all that exists
in me is castration does not matter because God, the
father, the analyst, the phallus do exist, not in me, but
in someone else who will eventually be capable of be-
stowing it on me. If the phallus does exist somewhere
in the Universe, then castration becomes incidental and
something to be overcome; and the omnipotence charged
on God shall be the surety of the omnipotence that in
my narcissism I consider mine." This is the reason I said
a while ago that what is transferred happens to be what
never existed and does not exist, is that which is not there
and is transferred onto the analyst, so that we can continue to believe that what doesn't exist in ourselves does
exist in someone else who will be part of ourselves.

II. A Vulnerable Point

One of the frequent discussions concerning transference evolves around the question of whether it is conscious or unconscious. There are certain psychoanalytic theories that speak of transference as something conscious. Other theories, to which I feel more akin, think that this is a phenomenon in which both the process and its consequence are unconscious. The patient believes that the analyst is—let us say—his or her father and not that it is as if the analyst were his or her father. Hence, what is working there is something equivalent to a symbolic equation. Therefore, it is always a process that in itself is basically psychotic, because transference requires this loss of reality judgment due to which the partner ceases to be considered as such and is transformed into that internal object that the patient projects. It is, therefore, a psychotic state. One object is taken for another. As if it were—and for the subject that enters a transferential relation, it is—another object. There is a loss of reality: the real object is unknown. There is also a psychotic restitution: the subject is delusional, and in his delusional states, as in the case of the mother suffering from Meynert's amentia, that the doll she is holding in her arms is her dead daughter. I don't think there can be any doubt about the psychotic nature of transference, if it really is a transference. It comes into existence through the unconscious mind's own way of working the primary process, by means of a dislodging or substitution. The fact that it is unconscious not only enables the primary process to start working (we know that this process could hardly function unless it looked away from reality and the real objects, since these would disavow and invalidate it) but is also a necessary condition for the transferred bond to continue existing. Becoming conscious would immediately imply a confrontation with reality, and it would be absolutely unthinkable for anyone, no matter which kind of logic he or she uses, to believe that Mauricio Abadi is Mauricio Abadi and Mr. N. N., the patient's father.

Anyway, it is true that the patient usually has a certain introspective knowledge that something strange is happening to him or her, but he or she doesn't know what. The feelings that invade the patient make him or her behave as if Mauricio Abadi were his or her father. But this is not equivalent to being aware of transference. It is merely perceiving facts about psychological life that are the consequence of a transference taking place with the patient's total unknowledge.

In conclusion, transference is an unconscious process. The patient might have enough information to know what is happening to him or her. But as Charcot said to Freud, "*Il y a savoir et savoir.*" ["There is knowledge and knowledge."]

And this intellectual knowledge has nothing to do with insight, with the direct knowledge that comes from living through the subjective experiences of a human being.

Yet, though that transference is unconscious and nobody really knows about his or her own transferring, the patient—and I mean especially the neurotic—perceives certain things that happen in his or her subjectivity that have to do with transference. The patient perceives them. So they are conscious. How do we explain this apparent contradiction?

III. The Two Transferences

I would like to explain now that what we call transference in the case of a neurotic is not really the same transference we have described up to now. Transference, as I proved earlier, is a psychotic phenomenon. Well then, what happens with this psychotic symptom in a neurotic personality? What I mean is, what happens with this delusional conviction that someone is the person he or she really is not? My answer is that the delusional conviction, the restitutive transference, is repressed. Because of repression it becomes unconscious, and yet it pushes, trying to become conscious. The flaws due to failures in the repression permit a return of the repressed, but on one condition. The one Freud taught us. A compromise with what would tend to keep it repressed. The result is a *Kompromisbildung*. A structure that is formed, among other things, by the delusional transference. Then, what appears in the preconscious is always a compromise; in it we recognize the particular transference we observe in neurotics.

There are therefore, in my judgment, two different types of transference, which we must differentiate. One of them is the transference proper, which we can observe in the psychotic patient, for whom the "other one" is nothing else than a distorting mirror in which he or she sees the reflection of a part of his or her own self or—what amounts to the same—the sediment of a previous libidinal relation to an object. The other transference is the one we see in the neurotic. In this case, we can suspect and *infer* that the true transference is repressed and unconscious, but what we can *see* is only a strange product (I know you are yourself, but despite my knowing this, for me, you are me), which shows the hybrid nature of every compromise structure. And what, if not a compromise structure, is a symptom? Therefore, what we call transference is, in the neurotic, nothing but a symptom. As Freud always clearly understood. Even though sometimes, in his texts, this conception can intermingle with the other one, which has more to do with psychosis, that different thing that is true transference. Still it is curious—paradoxes of the moment of discovery—that in the beginning Freud discarded the very existence of transference in psychosis (narcissistic neurosis), when it is precisely there that it exists. I think that these two transferences have to be distinguished from each other so as to avoid the confusion we are led to if we believe that transference is both conscious and unconscious. What happens—may I say it once more—is that true transference is unconscious and psychotic, and that the ill-termed neurotic transference is the product of a compromise, formed from what returned of the true transference from beyond repression, structured as a symptom. Even etymologically, symptom means coincidence. The relation between neurotic transference and true transference is only one of coincidence and of meaning. In other words it is something that points at something else that, being neurotics, we can never know in a direct way. We can only infer its existence and be content with this knowledge that results from a deduction. A neurotic patient says, "I know very well that you are not my father, I am not that crazy! I know that despite the fact that you are telling me that I am treating you as if you were the father I had in my childhood, I know for sure, let me tell you, that you are Dr. Abadi." When this patient tells me this, what he or she is letting me know is that his or her transference has been so repressed that he or she has achieved, not realizing his or her true mental reality, that I am his or her father. A repressed reality that has been substituted in the patient's conscious by the fiction that I am Dr. Abadi, to believe it is his or her neurosis. To think that Dr. Abadi for the patient can exist as something different from his or her father (Attention! not as something that carries the meaning of the father) is the patient's neurotic symptom. Then a technical corollary: to help the neurotic to gain awareness of his or her denied, repressed transference, and then to dissolve it through the destructuring interpretation of "false connections." To the contrary, with the psychotic, that part would be useless and avoidable, and the only thing to do is to attack and destroy the true transference through interpretation.

— 7 —

Reality and the Writer: Real Writing

Noé Jitrik

Many writers throughout the long history of Western culture have thought they could capture the secret of reality. Not its essence, which might seem philosophically reasonable, but its presence, just as it is, or, in other words, the structure, the meaning and purpose of things.

From the very beginning writers met with an obstacle, which we can consider as the first: "things" does not mean just some things; if they want to be coherent they would have to consider all things and everything. This difficulty, since it challenged their omnipotence, was always insurmountable, and this meant they had to choose a part; so they comfortably installed themselves in the use of "synecdoche." A part of a totality was presented as if it were the whole of that totality; thus they assumed that political matters meant the whole of reality, or this meaning was ascribed to certain social matters, or even certain questions of everyday life were taken to play that same part. They hardly ever admitted that it is impossible to arrive at an understanding of the totality of things with or without synecdoche.

Along with that difficulty, there is another one: What are things and what is their relation with what is real? Are they real because they are tangible things, or could there be something that not being a part of the material world of things could still be part of what is real? For example—a very far-fetched example—dreams, suppositions, the absurd products of imagination or thought. The more open-minded among these writers took for granted that these, too, were things and allowed them to live, in their writings, alongside the things they supposed to be real; as a consequence the scope of reality broadened but obviously left the task of answering these questions unresolved.

A second obstacle that we could consider is that to achieve this ambitious purpose we had and have no other instrument but words; as writers attempted to unveil the secret of reality, they could not help doing it with words, which in a strict sense are not of the same nature as things, though we readily admit that they are just as real as things. Putting it another way, when they wrote things, they assumed that in the writing those things appeared, so to speak, in their "thingness"; one is therefore entitled to think that not being able, even against their wishes, to give up words, they were disavowing them, denying their reality insofar as they pretended that through them they really made things appear; and if what is meant is reality, it is easy to conclude that the things evoked by words were, for them, more real than the words that evoked them and without which, of course, they would retain their secrecy.

As a matter of fact, what they thought they did was copy things with words; they supposed that they simply transcribed them, as if there were not two different sequences that touch each other, which they do, but which cannot intermingle, cannot penetrate each other. There was no other way for them but to represent things with words, which after all is something unavoidable, but for them that representation meant only the legitimation of what was being represented as a real thing.

The writers who thought this way, or whose way of writing evolved around this pretension of engulfing all or part of what is real, are known in the history of culture as realistic. They can be defined, restrictions included, by the above-mentioned notions; but if they knew and were aware of them, their intention was and is so powerful, so strongly ideological, that they could not accept them as a limitation. The realistic writer believes in what is usually called real; he has no doubts about it, nor does he question it, just as he has no doubt about his own capability to understand it, to enclose it, and to write it. He believes what his senses provide him with; he believes in what he understands about what he sees. At most, he may admit that reality reaches further than what he can see or understand immediately, or else that there might be aspects of things that are more real (less of an illusion?) than others, or in the case of the most sincere among them, that what is real is only what is at hand, what is touched and seen or personal experience, what is known from other people's experience—above all, if it is about knowledge, what has been written about it or what others have previously written about what they have seen or heard or known because they too have read it.

This means that the realistic writer, in a broad sense, also partly considers real what those (who through their writings teach him) have resolved about the relation between things and words.

But yet another equally difficult aspect to be considered remains: what we call things are not only individual objects, though they might as well be; above all, they are integrated systems, and because this is the way they work, they define what is empirically real. The world is, because diverse sets of elements form structures that have some meaning both in themselves and in their relation to the rest. One can speak of basic systems, of the natural system, of constituted systems, of the legal system, and so on, from the elemental to the most elaborate, like artistic or religious systems, to mention some. Therefore, what is real is systemic, and when writers attempt to represent it through writing, what they choose, believing they have grasped the key, is simply any one of those systems. What we have here is the return of the above-mentioned synecdoche; they choose only one system in order to write about the whole set of systems.

What immediately comes up at this point is another question: One supposes, one knows, that human beings of all epochs and places want or expect the diverse systems to work together harmoniously and to integrate into a superior system that includes them all; we can call it social or otherwise, but in any case it is that grand total that gives a meaning to all the summed-up parts. About that meaning, which is the meaning of a totality, there are divergent opinions and often strong differences. If all human beings agree that such a meaning must satisfy their primary needs and demands as well as their higher ones, without exception, there are still differences among them as to how to achieve this in a given place and time. Supposing that this meaning of the global system, on which there might be a general agreement, were invulnerable in its definition, it is very probable that some differences would exist concerning the answers that, each in its own realm, some of the lesser systems forming part of it offered; in this case, the discussion turns upon what is called injustice, oppression, distortion, lies, corruption, and so forth.

This can be read in an unavoidable way: each system has a value of its own, stemming both from the place it occupies with respect to the other systems and from the work required for its manufacture and maintenance. In turn, value is considered in relation to the meaning of the global system; there is some "minus value" in some of the systems, injustice, lies, oppression, inequality, and so on. This contrast generates a complementary activity, related to the question of value, termed *criticism*. No writer who wants to represent things will deprive himself or herself of doing it since, as we know, value is linked to expectations and ideals about the global system, which, as we also know, certain systems undo because of the way they work, at least in the view of those who observe them and try, through a representation, to uncover the secret of what is real, which is consequently betrayed.

Finally, we must consider another subject that comes up: the writer wants his or her writing to be something more than mere writing; he or she wants it to form part of a specific system and to acquire, within that system, a different meaning from that of the representation itself, independent of the things it represents. That system is called aesthetic, and by virtue of it, what is intended is that what is written have certain features that make it recognizable as an object, an act, or a work beyond a mere service to reality. Of course, the above-mentioned aesthetic system forms part of reality, but it is secondary to reality's other constituent parts. Its relation with them is not precise and not absolutely necessary for them; it is necessary only for those who believe that the secret of reality, values included, can be better disclosed with written words when these respond to that aesthetic system's own criteria; for some writers the aesthetic system exists per se, meaning that its value is not subordinated to the service it renders the representation.

Contrary to what was said at the beginning, right now it would seem as if these words about the relation between writers and reality describe not only many writers but all of them. It is not that way: the ones I have called realistic naturalize this rough plot and therefore not only are usually convinced that being realistic is something possible and feasible but also believe that precisely for that reason, they are doing, executing, the operation of putting that presence of real things into written words, in whatever system they choose to do it, even admitting the mentioned restrictions. Other authors give up the advantages of realism and choose a tangent, but even so they cannot ignore what they see, hear, and learn through reading. And though they understand that any approach to reality involves approaching the real words they operate with, they cannot give up or leave that universe of knowledge. I would call it the *Flaubert paradox*: "I want to write about nothing . . . ," he declared. I would add, "but I cannot, because words always signal a relation with things that cannot be over-looked."

Saying it otherwise: if words are signs, they contain a meaning without which the sign would be beheaded; precisely that meaning forms a bridge that reality builds toward the signs.

I would say that both groups, whether they know it or not, whether they want it or not, can only get closer to plain reality, via a detour, if they admit the reality of words, beyond the system that stands for it. Maybe this is what writers really do, beyond whatever they think or say they do or what some readers think writers do.

I am not saying this based on nothing; to start with, it is almost commonplace to say that literature reveals a society better than sociology itself. Marx himself said it, and perhaps that was why he gave literature power that his followers said they respected, though they did not necessarily completely understand it. Not paying attention to that recognition of literature, and consequently of the writers, in their attempt to unveil the secret of reality; on the opposite end of the spectrum, one often comes across the feeling, never feigned when the commitment is to realism, that literature is the great traitor of reality. Such a feeling is found not exclusively in readers but also in many writers. Perhaps this is what we hear in Pavese's last words, "a deed, enough of words."

Now, considering the way I have introduced the subject, and on the basis of some approximate conclusions I have arrived at, I could now introduce some new perspectives. For this, it suffices to formulate a new question, as follows: How do writers manage to write, be they candid believers in transcriptive representation or those who bet on what Mallarmé would have called "the tribe's" words?

To answer this question I will start by establishing a principle: what is characteristic to the writer is writing, and, therefore, whatever happens during the process of writing. This is why the process of writing is an object of psychoanalytic inquiry—because it is a mixture of sequences in diverse codes ranging from the cultural to the unconscious—beyond the question of intentionality, which would be a subject of general psychology. Consequently, from this point of view, it is hardly important whether the author intends to approach writing in this or in that way, or whether he or she believes or not in the existence of things. What the author cannot avoid is, as we already said, words, and how highly he or she esteems them is of no importance.

What is important is that the writer's universe of knowledge, originating in experience and in knowledge, and processed in his or her imagination, must be found and defined by his or her knowledge of words with the double purpose of erecting an aesthetic or symbolic realm, whichever you prefer to call it, where an autonomous meaning predominates, and another one that approaches the secret of what is real, even if it does not completely define it. The writer may do it simply because of a searching mind or a will to inquire; a pleasant feeling of reassurance; he or she is moved by an active ignorance, a spirit of adapting to what is visible; irritation about how what is visible seems to be organized; because of an intuition about what is beyond the visible; because of the belief that the visible and the invisible are one and the same thing; of the desire to promote a given cause; because of a critical clarity about the causes that appear to be protractions of the systems that build the global system.

Actually, this double purpose is an established fact and is the starting point of the writer's procedure. No

writer discusses it; he or she only operates, and does so
by first processing that universe of knowledge—his or her
own and other people's personal experience and knowledge acquired through reading—not to verify it or to
progress in his or her knowledge about himself or herself as an individual or in the objective knowledge about
things, but to be able to write it. Therefore, what is writ-
able must previously acquire a structure that the writer
must build; I call that previous structure the *referent*,
which is something like the image that will later lead to
the representation (for those who believe in it) or an *ex
nihilo* creation for those who would rather see it that way.

Consequently, what the writer writes is a referent
he or she previously built with the materials accessible
to him or her in two different but connected realms. The
first is the knowledge the writer has been accumulating
in direct, vivid relation with reality as he or she understands it, as it appears to him or her, and as he or she is
capable of working through it. The second one is the
knowledge of language which, in its constituents, implies
knowing about reality, because signs receive a necessary
flow of nutrition from reality, no matter how arbitrary
(as classic authors would have it) the relation between
reality and things may be. Language in motion processes
the first order of knowledge, takes it, models it, and
captures it, and the result of this work is a referent. It
always happens this way, but in the writer's case, the

only referents that matter are not all of them but only those that will enable him or her to write.

As you may notice, this assumes some preconditions: a certain wanting associated with some risk, and a social system that understands, admits, tolerates, and stimulates the production of the products that will result from that wanting. Here, the writer's so-called ethics appear; it is here that he or she chooses the way and the materials to build referents with the purpose of writing them.

From this derives the notion that this entire road can be predetermined; it actually seems to happen this way for the writers who define themselves as realistic. With the other writers, the road is more sinuous or tortuous, and this makes it harder to point out the process's diverse moments, the way every instance leads to transformations and displacements that are like plateaus or stages in the process of writing. However, this does not mean it is another road; what changes is the level of reality on which every decision is rooted and, therefore, on which idea of reality the writing is based.

The first one that comes to my mind, through analysis and experience, is exterioristic and evident or apparent; the second, I believe, tries to penetrate deeper layers, second levels in which reality's meaning shines in a different light, one that dazzles and blinds at the same time. What this implies is that because of writing, real-

ity changes, even if only because what is written is added
to reality, so that reality can no longer be seen as it was
seen before, even if it remains the same, its mystery
barely uncovered, its mystery still intact, ready to be
rewritten endlessly. This, I believe, is what this kind of
writer understands and does. As Macedonio Fernández
says, the writer makes reality, not realistic copies of it.

References

Abadi, M. (1960). *Renacimiento de Edipo* (*Rebirth of Oedipus*). Buenos Aires: Nova.
Ferrater Mora, J. (1965). *Diccionario de Filosofía* (*Dictionary
  of Philosophy*) vol. 2. Buenos Aires: Sudamericana.
Freud, S. (1899). Screen memories. *Standard Edition*
  3:301–322.
—— (1900). The interpretation of dreams. *Standard
  Edition* 4 and 5.
—— (1914). On narcissism: an introduction. *Standard
  Edition* 14:69–104.
—— (1937). Constructions in analysis. *Standard Edition*
  23:255–270.
Saint Augustine. (1984). *Confesiones* (*Confessions*). Libro
  11. Cap. 14. Buenos Aires: Paulinas.
Vernant, J.-P., and Vidal-Naquet, P. (1972). *Mythe et
  Tragédie en Grèce Ancienne.* (*Myth and Tragedy in
  Ancient Greece*). Paris: Gallimard.

Index

About the Authors

Mauricio Abadi, M.D., is a training analyst at the Argentine Psychoanalytical Association, of which he was formerly president. He is a full member of the International Psychoanalytical Association and in the practice of psychoanalysis in Buenos Aires, Argentina.

Susan Hale Rogers is a psychoanalyst in private practice in Buenos Aires, Argentina, and a member of the International Psychoanalytical Association as well as the Argentine Psychoanalytic Association.